HEARING INSTRUMENT

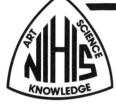

Selection and Evaluation

Edited by

Ernest Zelnick

Contributing Authors

Kenneth W. Berger
John K. Duffy
M. Duncan MacAllister
Geary McCandless
David A. Preves
Ernest Zelnick

Published by

National Institute for Hearing
Instruments Studies

Copyright © 1987
Library of Congress Catalog Card Number 87-60957

ZELNICK, Ernest (Editor)
HEARING INSTRUMENT SELECTION AND EVALUATION

Published by
National Institute for Hearing Instruments Studies,
Education Division of National Hearing Aid Society
20361 Middlebelt Road, Livonia, MI 48152
ISBN 0-934031-01-0
Manufactured in the United States of America

Preface

The main purpose of this textbook is to present in clear and concise terms the theory and procedures involved for several of today's most widely used hearing aid fitting methodologies. It is hoped that by reviewing each methodology the hearing aid specialist will achieve an enlightened position from which to practice.

An interesting consideration regarding the selection of hearing aids is the broad latitude the dispenser enjoys when applying amplification to the hearing loss. It is generally agreed that, for most hearing impairments, there is more than one way to obtain a successful fitting. Utilizing various response slopes, mold modifications, and circuit options the hearing aid specialist can approach the fitting in a number of ways and achieve verifiably positive results. Because of this flexibility in fitting methodology, it has often been said that our profession requires equal portions of art and science. In the pages that follow, the reader will be exposed to this fascinating blend of intuitive theory and scientific fact. It should be noted, however, that the information presented in this book is the opinion of the authors and not an endorsement by the National Institute for Hearing Instruments Studies.

In chapter one, Zelnick provides an historical overview of hearing aid selection procedures and explains which methods have gained wide acceptance. The psychoacoustic tests utilized for each method are given.

In chapter two, Zelnick continues by listing the various modes of amplification which are currently available. Although a strong proponent of binaural fittings, he indicates when the monaural fitting should be advised and issues guidelines for determining which ear should receive amplification. Special fitting such as CROS, BICROS, Y-Cord and Bone Conduction are discussed.

Chapter three is authored by Berger who describes his prescription method for hearing aid selection. This informative work includes an outline for hearing aid candidacy and steps for writing the hearing aid prescription. Fitting verification procedures are also covered.

In chapter four, McCandless acquaints the reader with the POGO method of instrument selection. His vast knowledge of the subject is readily apparent as he offers a convincing argument for the POGO rationale.

Chapter five is an illuminating introduction to the principles of Otometry. MacAllister does a masterful job of reporting on this unique methodology and its use of the damped wave train stimulus for hearing aid fitting measurements. The theory of Otometry and how it differs from other commonly used techniques is explained.

In the sixth chapter, Preves informs us of a fitting procedure which is rapidly growing in popularity. In his usual excellent fashion, he discusses the principles of insertion gain measurements and describes how use of the computer and probe microphone have made this practice possible.

In chapter seven, Duffy gives an outstanding presentation on sound field audiometry and hearing aid selection. His comparison of sound field data and computer probe tube measurements is thought provoking; and his discussion of acoustic phonetics should be mandatory reading for every hearing health professional.

As chairman of the National Institute for Hearing Instruments Studies, I would like to thank the authors for participating in this publishing project. Their contributions are immeasurable, as each author is either the originator or an acknowledged expert for the hearing aid selection procedure he has described. In addition, Dr. Ernest Zelnick, who served as Editor-in-Chief, must be congratulated for a job well done.

I wish to convey my respect and admiration for NIHIS Administrative Director Phyllis Wilson and the Institute board members. They are V. Hugh Bray, Jay H. Thurman, John H. Young, Jr., and Ernest Zelnick. These individuals unselfishly donated countless hours to the task of planning and coordinating the work on HEARING INSTRUMENT SELECTION AND EVALUATION. Without their professional foresight and commitment to excellence, this publication would not exist. Also, my sincere appreciation goes to NHAS President Richard ''Pat'' Clark and the Board of Governors for their unwaivering support of the Institute.

Michael K. Stone
Chairman

Foreword

The modern hearing aid is the most important rehabilitative instrument available for the treatment of the hearing-impaired. The rapid development of electronic circuitry and products during the last decade has made possible the miniaturization of high quality hearing aids. Hearing aids are now being produced which can automatically reduce low-frequency gain and filter steady state ambient noise. Multiband compression amplification is available for sensorineural hearing losses with narrow dynamic ranges. The suppression of acoustic feedback through the use of electronic circuits using adaptive notch and phase changing strategies will enable those with severe hearing-impairments to take advantage of miniaturization. It appears that the engineers and manufacturers of hearing aids have done their job well. It now becomes the responsibility of the hearing aid specialist to apply such engineering marvels to appropriate hearing aid fittings.

The National Hearing Aid Society and the National Institute for Hearing Instruments Studies (NIHIS), aware of the tremendous importance of the methodology of hearing aid selection have supported the preparation and publication of this first textbook entirely devoted to hearing aid selection and evaluation.

A review of the literature as I explained in chapter I indicates that professionals involved in hearing aid selection have not been able to agree or accept any one suggested method for selecting an appropriate hearing aid. Therefore, it was decided by the Board of the National Institute for Hearing Instruments Studies that those proposed procedures that were being used by most specialists for selecting a hearing aid would be described in detail by their advocates.

I wish to thank the authors who contributed so much to this textbook. I also want to thank the past Chairman of the Institute Board (NIHIS) Richard L. Clark, for his personal support of this undertaking. I further wish to thank the present members of the NIHIS Board, Chairman Michael K. Stone, V. Hugh Bray, Jay H. Thurman, John H. Young, Jr., and Phyllis V. Wilson, Administrative Director of the Board, for their critical review and suggestions.

I must thank my wife Harriet, and my office staff for their tireless help on this project, and my sincere thanks to all of the members of the National Hearing Aid Society for inviting me to speak at national and state conventions on the subject of hearing aid selection which created the desire in me to formulate the current proposals in this textbook in Chapters I and II.

I now commend this book to all who believe as I do that every effort must be made not only to design better instruments of amplification, but also better procedures must be developed for the selection and assessment of appropriate hearing aid performance characteristics for the enhancement of communicative abilities of the hearing impaired of our Society.

Ernest Zelnick, Ph.D.
Editor

LIST OF CONTRIBUTING AUTHORS

Kenneth W. Berger, Ph.D.	Professor Emeritus in Audiology, Kent State University, Kent, Ohio
John K. Duffy, Ph.D.	Professor Emeritus in Audiology, Brooklyn College, City University of New York, Brooklyn, New York
M. Duncan MacAllister, Ph.D.	President, Emtech Laboratories, Inc., Roanoke, Virginia
Geary McCandless, Ph.D.	Professor of Audiology, Department of Communication Disorders, The University of Utah, Salt Lake City, Utah
David A. Preves, Ph.D.	Vice President, Research and Design, Argosy Electronics, Edina, Minnesota
Ernest Zelnick, Ph.D.	President of Professional Hearing Aids, Brooklyn, New York

CONTENTS

V. PRINCIPLES OF OTOMETRY
M. Duncan MacAllister

VI. APPLICATION OF PROBE MICROPHONES FOR VALIDATING HEARING AID FITTINGS
David A. Preves

VII. SOUND FIELD AUDIOMETRY AND HEARING AID SELECTION
John K. Duffy

1

REVIEW OF SUGGESTED HEARING AID PROCEDURES

ERNEST ZELNICK

INTRODUCTION

Since about 1904, hearing aids have been dispensed in the United States
and there are probably more than three million people in this country
now wearing some form of amplification. Most studies have indicated
that the preponderence of hearing aid users are satisfied with the
instrumentation furnished to them. However, over the years there have
been proposals made in order to obtain maximum benefit for the user
from the hearing aid selected. Fifty years ago, in 1937, Robert West
in the "Rehabilitation of Speech" suggested a procedure of 'mirroring
the audiogram' for proper amplification. Over the years, many other
procedures have appeared in the professional literature for hearing aid
selection. This book published by the National Institute for Hearing
Instruments Studies will acquaint hearing aid dispensers with current
methodology for hearing aid evaluation and selection. Since the method
of selecting a specific hearing aid and earmold for a particular hearing
loss remains one of the most controversial aspects of the rehabilitation
programs for the hearing-impaired, the chapters of this book will
represent different procedures. Every attempt has been made to have

the leading advocate of a particular methodology of hearing aid selection write a chapter and argue his position. Therefore, it is the hope of the editor that a reading of this textbook will enable dispensers to supplement their particular office protocol, thereby resulting in additional benefits to hearing aid users.

Most contemporary professionals involved in hearing aid selection attempt to recommend amplification containing performance characteristics based on psychoacoustic (behavioral) data. There are proposals for the determination of the gain-frequency characteristic of an appropriate hearing aid, based on thresholds of hearing. Other writers have suggested that such characteristic be based on either most comfortable loudness level or comfortable loudness contours. Almost all procedures for hearing aid selection suggest that the maximum pressure output of the aid does not exceed the threshold of discomfort. Therefore, every effort must be made by the specialist in conducting audiometric testing to insure the reliability and validity of audiometric responses. The procedure adopted for obtaining the required audiometric data should consider the duration of such tests. Many geriatric clients have short attention spans and become easily fatigued, which can affect the validity of responses. Care should be exerted in the selection of word lists for speech audiometry, as a short list of words, although convenient for the tester, can prove unreliable on retest. Instructions to the client being tested should be explicit, simple and understandable. Audiometric equipment must be calibrated and tested for accuracy periodically.

The performance characteristic of the hearing aid selected can be measured in test boxes using 2cc couplers to ascertain whether or not the gain, frequency response and maximum pressure output conform to the specifications published by the hearing aid manufacturer. In fact, those hearing aid specialists who prefer probe tube microphone measurements can obtain the actual electroacoustic responses of the selected aid at the eardrum.

Any method of hearing aid selection adopted by specialists is only as effective as the accuracy of the audiometric profile to which it is applied. Therefore, competence is desired at every stage of the testing procedure as well as the application of methodology to select those performance characteristics of hearing aids to meet the audiometric needs of the client.

Assessment of the hearing aid selected must be a part of any hearing aid evaluation procedure. Many suggestions for testing the performance of a hearing aid worn by the user are proposed in this textbook. It is my opinion that hearing aids should be evaluated based on the listener's auditory performance. I have therefore, stressed the importance of both pure-tone and speech soundfield audiometry as a method of assessing the real-ear performance of the client with the specific hearing aid.

Chapter Objectives

The purpose of this chapter is to review the literature on methodology for hearing aid selection and assessment. From Fletcher (1926) who described materials for the evaluation of hearing aids, Knudsen and Jones (1936) who suggested the use of speech testing for evaluating benefits of a hearing aid and West (1937) who proposed 'mirroring the audiogram' numerous procedures have emerged over the past sixty years for selecting and evaluating the effectiveness of hearing aids. The object of this particular chapter is to acquaint hearing aid dispensers with those procedures that have been most widely applied. Especially, those methods of hearing aid evaluation which have attained acceptance by many specialists are explained and discussed.

The psychoacoustic tests required under each method of hearing aid selection are listed and described. The electroacoustic performance characteristics proposed by various writers to achieve maximum speech intelligibility under each particular method are discussed. Therefore it is the intention of this author to furnish the reader with a background of the various philosophical considerations involved in the rationale of a procedure. Studies and articles which have elucidated weaknesses as to reliability and validity of a suggested methodology are also mentioned so that the reader can properly assess the value of its application in their own office protocol. Perhaps, this chapter will enable a dispenser to select a portion of a particular procedure and add to his own method of selection.

Methods of hearing aid selection have been classified into five categories; prescriptive, comparative, subjective, objective and combined procedures. An object of this chapter is to acquaint hearing aid professionals with the various proposed methodology for selecting appropriate hearing aids. The current trend appears to be the use of the prescriptive methods by most hearing aid specialists. The most widely accepted prescriptive procedures are presented and merits as well as shortcomings of suggested methods for selecting hearing aids are explained.

A further object of this chapter was to present to the hearing aid specialist criteria for acceptance of a suggested procedure for hearing aid selection which could serve as a guideline for use of all or a part of a proposed methodology. It is hoped that creative dispensers can modify their own procedures for the selection and recommendation of hearing aids so that greater benefit can be achieved on the part of the user.

The hearing aid selected by any procedure should be assessed for its performance by real-ear testing. This chapter suggests the use of pure-tone sound field audiometry together with speech recognition tests using phonemic scoring as a method of validation.

REVIEW OF SUGGESTED METHODS OF HEARING AID SELECTION

Historically, the first suggestion for fitting hearing aids in accordance with psychoacoustic data obtained from the hearing-impaired individual appeared in the mid-thirties. In fact, West (1937) in the Rehabilitation of Speech encouraged selective amplification based on the thresholds of hearing.

A review of the literature on hearing aid selection indicates three main proposals in the early period of hearing aid evaluation. These early methods of selecting hearing aids were supported mainly by hearing aid manufacturers and were employed by the preponderance of hearing aid dispensers. The hearing aid was normally selected based on the client's audiometric profile. The audiometric information consisted of the following:

1 Thresholds of hearing — air and bone
   The audiogram furnished the dispenser with the information as to the severity of the loss, the configuration of the hearing loss and whether the loss is conductive, sensorineural or mixed.

2 Speech discrimination scores
   This information enables the dispenser to select the ear to be fitted in monaural recommendations and also some predictability as to how well the client can be expected to perform with the use of amplification.

3 Comfortable loudness
   a. Most comfortable loudness level
      Several procedures have been proposed for raising the average level of speech to the most comfortable loudness level of the ear fitted.
   b. Equal loudness contours
      This procedure suggests determining the most comfortable loudness level at 1000Hz and then obtaining an equal loudness contour through a matching technique at other critical frequencies.

4 Threshold of discomfort
   Most suggested procedures for hearing aid evaluation stress the importance of the maximum pressure output of the hearing aid not exceeding the threshold of discomfort (TD).

The hearing aid selected should have the specific performance characteristics in terms of gain, frequency response and maximum pressure output in accordance with the psychoacoustic profile based on hearing threshold levels, most comfortable loudness level and threshold of discomfort. The frequency response configuration was selected based on the slope of the audiogram for the ear fitted. The three early prescriptive procedures for selecting hearing aids were:

   A. Mirroring the audiogram

   B. Equal-loudness contour

   C. Bisection

A. *Mirroring the Audiogram Procedure*

This method, based on having the frequency-gain characteristic of a hearing aid mirror the hearing loss as indicated on the pure-tone air conduction audiogram, was first described by West (1937). It was an attempt to select the hearing aid which would provide sufficient amplification to compensate for the loss shown by the audiogram. This method of providing gain to mirror the audiogram was very effective for the large number of persons with conductive hearing losses who sought hearing aid help prior to the advent of middle ear surgery. However, for those suffering from sensorineural hearing loss, a strict mirroring of the audiogram could result in excessive amplification because of recruitment and limited dynamic ranges. Individuals suffering from sensorineural hearing loss due to cochlear dysfunction normally experience the phenomena of recruitment, which is the abnormal growth of loudness with linear increase in intensity. In addition, the threshold of discomfort for people with sensorineural losses may even be lower than the threshold of discomfort of the normal ear. Therefore, there is a much smaller dynamic range in which sound pressure can be comfortably tolerated than in the normal ear.

Supporters of 'mirror imaging' such as Pascoe (1975) suggest that the frequency response mirror the sound field audiogram but are not necessarily recommending gain equal to the hearing loss because of the recruitment factor. Duffy and Zelnick (1985) recommend a mirroring approach to selection of appropriate hearing aid performance characteristics but again, not seeking to overcome the hearing loss by the gain of the aid but rather an attempt to mirror the slope of the audiogram. Their concern is with the relationship of gain at one frequency to the gain at other critical frequencies for speech intelligibility. Overall gain can be controlled by the volume control of the particular hearing aid (most hearing aids have a range of at least 30dB in terms of overall gain). However, the relationship of gain at various frequencies, important for processing speech, cannot be controlled significantly in most commercial hearing aids. Therefore, it is the function of the professional involved in hearing aid selection, to recommend the aid which has a frequency response which will produce maximum audibility for the speech spectrum. The modern concept of mirroring the audiogram really involves the provision of amplification in relation to the shape or slope of the particular audiogram. The high-frequency sounds (consonants) important for the understanding of speech must be made audible by providing amplification in this frequency area (1500Hz-6500Hz) at sensation levels of at least 20dB above the threshold of hearing of the impaired ear. Low-frequency sounds of speech (mostly vowels), where many people with sensory (cochlear) hearing losses have better hearing sensitivity, require less amplification.

The pattern of amplification thus provided should result in a response which approximates the equal loudness contours for speech at supra-threshold levels. Proponents of mirror imaging claim that output limiting circuitry and compression amplification available in commercial hearing aids enable the dispenser to provide sufficient amplification in the high-frequency regions without exceeding thresholds of discomfort.

B. *Equal-Loudness Contour Procedure*
Among the first supporters of the principle of determining most comfortable loudness for the purpose of hearing aid selection were Watson and Knudsen (1940). They claimed that the optimum hearing aid performance could be obtained by amplifying the average level of speech to the most comfortable equal-loudness contour of the hearing-impaired ear. The method requires that the most comfortable level for a 1000Hz tone be obtained for the hearing-impaired subject. Then through a loudness matching procedure the intensity required at other significant specific frequencies such as 250Hz, 500Hz, 2000Hz and 4000Hz, thus obtaining the subject's comfortable equal-loudness contour. The frequency response of the recommended hearing aid should mirror the difference between the subject's equal-loudness contour and the auditory threshold. Again, the concern is with the relative gain and not the absolute gain which the user of the hearing aid can control through the volume control. Watson and Knudsen reported much better speech discrimination scores when using their method for relative gain or shaping of the frequency response than when using other frequency-gain characteristics. Despite good results obtained by use of the equal-loudness contour procedure, most specialists involved in hearing aid selection have not adopted this technique. The reason Watson and Knudsen's procedure never attained wide acceptance is probably due to the fact that the method is unduly time consuming for clinical application. In

addition, many difficult-to-test subjects find loudness matching too sophisticated a task.

Markle and Zaner (1966) stated that since a hearing aid affects the auditory stimulus rather than the auditory threshold, the fact that a sensorineural ear recruits (abnormal growth of loudness) should be considered in selecting the gain characteristic of a hearing aid. They included in their article a laddergram illustrating a case of abnormally rapid loudness increment and the gain that would be required for the particular ear with a 40dB HL loss, for soft speech (35dB), for average speech (50dB) and for loud speech (65dB HL) (it should be mentioned that speech levels are usually referenced to SPL, see Figure 1).

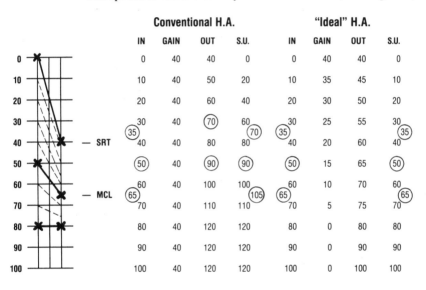

N.B. The above is based on the assumption that recruitment is linear and is complete at 80 db.

Fig. 1. A laddergram illustrating a hypothetical case of abnormally rapid loudness increment. The hearing loss for speech (SRT) is 40 dB.

Explanation of Figure 1.

The S.U. column in above illustration by Markle and Zaner refers to speech understanding or how sound intensity is experienced by the listener. Actually it is equal loudness for speech of impaired-ear compared to the normal ear. At an output of 70 dB into the impaired-ear using a conventional hearing aid, the loudness would be perceived equal to the sound pressure at 60 dB in the normal ear. With the use of the ideal hearing aid, an output of 80 dB and above would be perceived in the impaired-ear at the same loudness as in the normal ear. This illustration indicates that no further amplification is required once recruitment is complete in an impaired-ear.

The circled 35 dB input represents soft speech, the circled 50 dB input represents average speech and the circled 65 dB HL input represents loud speech.

Therefore, overall gain of a hearing aid should be based on most comfortable loudness levels and not on threshold levels. For a sensorineural hearing loss the most comfortable loudness level takes the recruitment factor of the ear into account and since recruitment is not always linear and changes with frequency and with the ear involved, basing the overall gain on threshold levels would ignore this important factor.

Zelnick (1982) has proposed the use of most comfortable loudness (MCL) level for speech as the criteria for overall gain and has suggested the following formulae:

Average HAIC gain = MCL + 20dB-65dB + 10dB
Average HF gain = MCL + 20dB-55dB + 10dB
Reference test gain (RTG) = MCL + 20dB-55dB

The 20dB is a correction factor to convert the most comfortable loudness level (MCL) measured with the audiometer in dB HL to dB SPL. The average level of speech is 65dB SPL.

The average HAIC gain is based on measurements made at 500Hz, 1000Hz and 2000Hz. The 10dB is added in the formulae above so that the aid is not worn at full-gain setting of the volume control when the aid is adjusted to a preferred listening level by the user.

The average HF gain and reference testing is based on measurements made at 1000Hz, 1600Hz and 2500Hz. The 10dB is added in the average HF gain formula so that the aid is not worn at maximum setting of the volume control, as explained above.

One should be aware that in everyday use, the client will determine the gain setting of the aid in keeping with his/her needs and comfort.

C. *Bisection Procedure*

Among the earliest methods for selecting the frequency-gain characteristics of a hearing aid was the bisection method. This procedure, as proposed by Wallenfels (1967), was an attempt to amplify speech to the mid-level of the dynamic range (threshold of discomfort minus speech reception threshold) of the impaired ear. Actually, Wallenfels recommended the optimum hearing level curve be equal to the line of bisection in the region of 1000Hz to 4000Hz. Above 4000Hz, he suggests that for a narrow dynamic range, the hearing level curve be closer to the threshold curve. Below 1000Hz, if the slope of the line of bisection is steep then the hearing level curve continues downward with the same degree of slope. However, if the slope of the line of bisection between 1000Hz and 4000Hz is less than 8dB per octave, then the hearing level curve is given a downward slope of 8 to 10dB per octave below 1000Hz. This suggestion is made by Wallenfels in order to limit the amount of amplification in the low-frequency area, and thus avoid any masking effect of low-frequency components of speech on the high-frequencies. The suppression of low-frequencies also prevents over-amplification of ambient noise which is often low-frequency in character and most disturbing to many hearing aid users.

To my knowledge, no research has been conducted to verify the assumption of bisection adherents that the halfway level of the dynamic range of the impaired ear is a level for maximum speech intelligibility. It would appear that better user benefits can be obtained by providing amplification of the average level of speech to a most comfortable loudness level.

Comparative Procedures

Carhart (1946) described a comparative procedure based on speech audiometry for hearing aid selection which was widely used with hearing-impaired veterans of World War II, and for many years after. In fact, even today it is still widely employed in many academic and clinical settings. The intent of this approach is to select the best hearing aid from a group of hearing aids chosen for the test. The criteria for selecting the hearing aid which Carhart believed would provide maximum benefit for a hearing-impaired client are as follows:

(1) effective gain, the greatest improvement in speech reception threshold (unaided speech reception threshold compared to aided speech reception threshold).

(2) the best word discrimination score (PB-50's at sensation level of 25dB above SRT).

(3) tolerance limit.

(4) efficiency in a background of noise (the ability to maintain satisfactory speech discrimination in the highest level of noise).

Carhart stressed that the measurements obtained would help to identify any problem that the client may have in the use of the hearing aid. Each of the four criteria is tested separately. Selection of the hearing aid is made sometimes in terms of one criterion, and sometimes in terms of several criteria. Many professionals still using the Carhart procedure prefer to give the greatest weight to the word discrimination score.

The comparative procedure does not attempt to correlate psychoacoustic data obtained for an individual to the electroacoustic performance characteristic of a hearing aid. The comparative procedure relies rather on speech audiometry in making a decision on which the hearing aid accomplishes maximum benefit for the hearing-impaired.

It is interesting to note that Carhart recommended that the presentation level for speech discrimination testing of PB 50's be at a sensation level of 25dB above SRT, with the aid adjusted to reach a most comfortable loudness level. Many professionals employing the Carhart procedure have modified the speech discrimination test by presenting PB words or other word lists at a fixed level of 40dB to 50dB HL (60dB to 70dB SPL). This presentation level appears to have more merit, in that the input speech level in assessing the relative performance of various hearing aids is the level closer to average conversational speech. Millin (1980) has aptly explained the advantage of using a constant stimulus level (modified Carhart procedure), because it permits the aid to function more as it would in everyday use, and increases the sensitivity of word discrimination tests to differences in hearing aid frequency response effects.

The reliability of traditional hearing aid evaluation by the Carhart procedure was seriously questioned as a result of a study by Shore, Bilger and Hirsh (1960). Their study ranked the relative effectiveness of a number of hearing aids which differed significantly in electroacoustical performance characteristics. The research indicated large variations in test-retest scores for different hearing aids, settings and days. In fact, they concluded:

> "that the reliability of these measures is not good enough to warrant the investment of a large amount of clinical time with them in selecting hearing aids."

There has probably been some over-generalization from the conclusions made by Shore and his associates in their study, which has lead to their study being used as a reference for the position that all comparative hearing aid evaluation procedures are unnecessary and unreliable. It should therefore be pointed out that the Shore et al. study did not actually use the procedure suggested by Carhart. It differed from Carhart's method in the following ways:

1. Carhart had recommended using the full 50-word list (PB50) whereas the Shore et al. study used half-word lists of 25 words. Use of a smaller sample of words will affect the reliability of speech audiometry as reported by Raffin and Thorton (1980).

2. Carhart suggested that the presentation level for speech discrimination testing be 25dB above the aided speech reception threshold whereas Shore and his associates presented the monosyllabic words at a 40dB sensation level above SRT. This presentation level of 40dB may have been too intense for the sensorineural group they tested and could cause a diminishment of speech discrimination in the impaired ear. Scharf and Florentine (1982) have reported that spectral resolution

decreases in both normal and sensorineural-impaired ears at high sound pressure levels. In fact, the use of amplification by hearing-impaired listeners results in speech being delivered at higher sound pressure levels to these individuals than to normal hearing persons. Therefore, presentation levels should be at minimum sensation levels sufficient for attaining maximum speech intelligibility. Most specialists using a comparative procedure today, would prefer a constant presentation level of from 40dB HL to 50dB HL (60dB-70dB SPL) and a setting of the hearing aid at a most comfortable loudness level. As a result of the Shore et al. study some clinical professionals advocated the abandonment of comparative hearing aid selection. Resnick and Becker (1963) suggested that the traditional Carhart procedure was based on three basic assumptions:

1 That there are significant differences existing among hearing aids as reflected in the user's ability to understand everyday speech.

2 That these observed differences among aids change and vary between users of hearing aids and that there is an interaction between people and hearing aids.

3 That these differences existing between hearing aids can be measured reliably by monosyllabic word (PB50) intelligibility scores.

Other writers on comparative procedures for hearing aid selection have suggested an additional two premises:

4 That the relative performance of listeners tested with a number of hearing aids will remain stable over a period of time.

5 That the performance of a client with a specific hearing aid is predictive of the patient's performance in everyday life. Efforts have been made by researchers over the years to validate the above assumptions since comparative procedures for selecting hearing aids would not be justified should such assumptions be proven false.

What appears obvious to many dispensers, that there are significant differences among hearing aids as they affect listener's speech performance, has been difficult to verify. Studies comparing speech discrimination scores with different hearing aids have not yielded significant differences unless performance characteristics are selected which would be inappropriate for a particular audiogram (Schwartz and Walden 1980). It would appear that the failure to find significant differences in speech scores is probably due to the use of speech material as testing signals which are insensitive to the fine differences accruing from changes in electroacoustic performance characteristics of hearing aids. Zelnick (1970) indicated that the use of phonemic scoring in speech discrimination testing as advocated by Duffy (1967), using

Peterson and Lehiste revised CNC lists (1962), provided a more sensitive measure than the use of the 50 PB word lists with scores computed on an all-or-nothing correct basis (Duffy will elaborate on the use of phonemic scoring and furnish new word lists that he has prepared in chapter VII).

The fact that many professionals are still involved in comparative hearing aid evaluation procedures is evidence that they are still convinced that there are significant differences among hearing aids which are reflected in the client's performance in communication in every day life. Research is continuing in the search for speech stimuli which will provide more sensitive measures of evaluating hearing aid performance and giving better predictability as to how the user will perform in everyday life experiences.

Zerlin (1962) reported a study which indicated that quality judgments were more efficient predictors of hearing aid performance than were intelligibility scores achieved with monosyllabic words when tested in quiet. However, judgments of quality are not necessarily conclusive as to the performance of a hearing aid in terms of speech intelligibility. Probably, a multidimensional test of both intelligibility for speech as well as the quality of sound will emerge for assessment of the aid which will furnish optimum performance. In this respect, most professionals are no longer looking for the best aid but rather for an appropriate hearing aid for a particular client Carhart (1950). The clinician cannot continue to search indefinitely for the best hearing aid fitting or the ultimate in terms of speech intelligibility but rather select a number of hearing aids having performance characteristics based on the audiometric profile and from them, using proper evaluation techniques (preferably sound field audiometry), choose the aid that appears to give the best audibility, speech intelligibility, comfortability and quality of sound in meeting the client's needs.

It has been demonstrated by Olsen and Wilber (1967) that the use of a competing signal with monosyllabic word tests can measure performance differences in varying amplification systems. Other studies have also arrived at the same conclusion; that testing speech recognition in backgrounds of noise results in differences in understanding as a function of amplification system differences that are not evidenced in testing speech discrimination in quiet. However, the reliability on re-test of speech discrimination in a background of noise is still poor unless the partial scoring method is employed. I normally use a signal-to-noise ratio of +5dB in testing sensorineural hearing losses in a sound field.

The second assumption; that there is an interaction between the hearing aid and the user has also been difficult to prove. This assumption negates any conclusion that there is 'a best hearing aid' which will be appropriate for all hearing-impaired with similar audiograms. In fact, many individuals with similar audiograms indicate significant differences in real ear response when fitted with the same hearing aid. Since there is an interactive effect between a particular hearing aid and a user, response from hearing aids have to be compared by real-ear sound field tests as to the benefits derived.

The Harvard Report (Davis et al. 1947) which concluded that selective amplification was "wasteful of time and effort" recommended that hearing aids have either a flat response or a high-frequency emphasis of 6dB rise per octave. Fortunately, hearing aid manufacturers generally ignored the report's findings and recommendations and continued to design hearing aids with various frequency responses and incorporated tone controls for frequency modification. Subsequent research and investigations has discredited the conclusions of the Harvard Report as will be discussed by Duffy, in detail, in chapter VII.

The third assumption of comparative hearing aid selection procedures; that differences can be demonstrated reliably by the use of monosyllabic word scores has been questioned by the Shore et al. study. As mentioned previously for speech discrimination scores to furnish statistically reliable results much larger word lists would have to be employed. In order to attain the predicted accuracy that we desire, the number of words would have to be increased to such extent that a very great deal of time would be required. Such lengthy testing would be fatiguing and clearly impractical in a clinical setting. Therefore, specialists involved in comparative hearing aid selection methodology have changed this assumption to one that can be validated. The modified assumption states that these differences among hearing aids can be demonstrated by tests comparing the aid, such as pure-tone sound field, speech audiometry with phonemic scoring, insertion gain, judgments of intelligibility and judgments of quality. This modified assumption has been proven true. Differences existing among hearing aids have been reliably demonstrated by the use of sound field audiometry using 5% warbled pure-tones (see chapter VII on sound field audiometry by Duffy).

The assumption of relative performance remaining stable over time appears to be valid for tests conducted in a sound field using warbled pure-tones. Sound field testing performed for many years in the office of the author of this chapter has shown results to be quite stable and reliable over time. Watson and Knudson wrote in 1940 that speech discrimination score test results depended strongly on exposure time and training. More recently, Schwartz and Walden (1983) reported that there was large variability in word recognition scores in noise in some patients when tested over a five day period. Again, this result could be due in some degree to the variability of speech discrimination testing when scored with an all-or-nothing correct method. Phonemic scoring appears to be not only a more sensitive measure but also results in less variability and better reliability. Those advocating the use of speech audiometry in comparative hearing aid selection also suggest a period of adaptation and training with the aid and then re-testing for speech recognition ability.

The last assumption of predictability of a client's performance in everyday life with a given hearing aid based on the listener's performance with the aid in the clinical testing situation has been the most difficult to prove. There are so many acoustic variables in everyday listening that affect the user's performance with a recommended hearing aid that it has been most difficult for the dispenser to predict actual benefit. Suggestions have been made that the individual be tested in an environment that more closely simulates the acoustic environment to be encountered by the client. However, hearing-impaired people live and work in different surroundings and it is impossible to structure a testing environment that is similar to the acoustic signals that a particular subject will experience. The hearing aid specialist has the responsibility of selecting a hearing aid appropriate for the hearing-impaired ear. The hearing aid in meeting the needs of the client should have the necessary controls to modify the response of the aid under changing acoustical conditions.

Governmental inquiries into hearing aid selection and dispensing in the 1970's indicated the need for more intensive research in this discipline. Many of the studies from the early 1970's to date have stressed the importance of real-ear measurements in hearing aid selection. Unfortunately, with a few exceptions, past research has not taken account of relevant acoustic effects in their description of frequency-gain characteristics of hearing aids used in their studies. The stated performance characteristics of hearing aids were often nominal and could be used only for relative measurements. As acoustical factors affecting hearing aid performance were investigated and became better understood, the importance of real-ear measurements became critical. Therefore, current methodology of hearing aid selection is concerned with the appropriate characteristics of amplification and methods of validation of the effectiveness of the amplifier when used with a customized earmold.

CURRENT PRESCRIPTIVE PROCEDURES

In the 1970's there was increased research in hearing aid acoustics. In the Scandinavian countries, there were a number of excellent papers on the effects of earmolds on the acoustic performance of hearing aids. In the United States, there were inquiries as to both selection procedures as well as to methods of distribution of hearing aids by congressional committees, the Federal Trade Commission and the Food and Drug Administration. One of the results of these governmental hearings was the realization that most of the hearing aid selective procedures could not be substantiated by scientific investigations. There were many suggested procedures for selection of hearing aids and many clinicians and dispensers had their own favorite method of determining the appropriate hearing aid. The time was ripe for a scientific approach to the art of hearing aid selection.

It appeared necessary to many specialists in hearing aid selection that the alternative approach was one which would make the hearing aid recommendation dependent on real-ear measurements. Since the ultimate goal of a hearing aid is to improve speech perception for hearing-impaired listeners, it would be necessary to have data on the amplification characteristics of a hearing aid in relation to the hearing-impairment. The selection of the appropriate frequency-gain characteristic for a hearing aid has been the subject of intensive research. Dugal, et al. (1980) have written concerning this problem:

> "The optimum choice of frequency-gain characteristic is likely to depend on interactions between properties of the sound source (e.g. the speech of men, women and children typically have different spectra and amplitude distributions), the transmission channel (which may be noisy and reverberant and which may introduce nonlinear distortions), and the receiver (i.e., the details of the hearing loss and the preferred listening level) —"

Although the above writers feel that the determination of the appropriate frequency-gain characteristic is a very difficult problem, this author and others involved in this discipline do not feel that it is as formidable as they have described it. On the contrary, many procedures have been suggested and some will be described in the chapters of this book for determining appropriate electroacoustic performance characteristics of hearing aids.

It appears that the current methodology for hearing aid selection employed by most clinicians and dispensers adheres to the principle of basing the selection on real-ear measurements. Unfortunately, some of the proposed real-ear methods are pseudo-real-ear and should be described correctly. However, in order to formulate a method of hearing aid selection that could be universally accepted and adopted for achieving maximum intelligibility and comfortability the following criteria should apply:

CRITERIA FOR PRESCRIPTIVE PROCEDURE FOR HEARING AID SELECTION

1 The required performance characteristics of the hearing aid recommended should be based on psychoacoustic data from

audiometric evaluation for hearing aids (e.g. thresholds of hearing, most comfortable loudness levels, thresholds of discomfort and speech discrimination scores).

2 The procedure should be relatively simple to conduct.

3 The time required for the conduction of audiometric and electroacoustic tests should be as brief as possible (people become fatigued with lengthy testing and results are unreliable).

4 A suggested procedure should be based on sound and proven principles of acoustics (it should be scientific and not intuitive).

5 The results of the suggested procedure should be verifiable (the procedure should include some rationale for assessing the results).

6 The suggested procedure should not require very highly specialized and costly equipment (the equipment suggested should be easy to operate and function efficiently).

7 The suggested procedure should be applicable to all subjects and groups, regardless of age, language or education (it should apply to difficult-to-test subjects).

The editor of this book encourages the reader to check the above guidelines for a proposed procedure for hearing aid selection as he reads the following chapters and decide which of these suggested methods meets all or most of the above criteria.

HIGH FREQUENCY EMPHASIS

Most of us, concerned with appropriate hearing aid amplification, have adhered to the position that the gain of the aid should increase in frequency regions where the hearing loss is more severe. Selective amplification is the attempt to select electroacoustic characteristics of the aid based on the audiometric data of the patient with the goal of achieving maximum speech perception and comfort. In accordance with this principle of selective amplification, most hearing aids are recommended which have frequency responses accentuating the high-frequencies for the following reasons:

1 Most sensorineural hearing losses have audiograms which indicate greater loss of hearing in the higher frequencies and therefore require greater amplification in this frequency area.

2 Earmolds normally occlude the ear canal, thus destroying the natural high-frequency resonance of the external ear (this resonance is normally about 2700Hz).

3 The intensity of the high-frequency components of the speech spectra is approximately 15dB to 30dB lower than the low-frequency components of average speech (greater amplification is therefore required in the high-frequency area in order to make this frequency area of speech audible).

4 Ambient environmental noise normally is predominantly low-frequency in composition and a hearing aid is normally recommended which limits amplification in the low-frequency area in order to suppress such annoying background noise.

Although most current hearing aid methodology agrees with the principle of selective amplification, various proposals suggest different formulae for determining the actual frequency-gain characteristics of an appropriate hearing aid. Recent research has concluded that selective amplification does result in a more appropriate hearing aid selection and the preponderance of recommendations by professionals in this discipline are based on the audiometric profile of the hearing-impaired person. However, differences among methods of selection do exist. In fact, the controversy over procedure and instrumentation to be employed in hearing aid selection has intensified. As different viewpoints are expressed and new methodology proposed and defended in the literature on hearing aid selection, the problems in achieving a science of hearing aid evaluation become better understood and closer to solution. It is evident to the editor of this book that further research is required in audiometric testing, in electroacoustic testing of the hearing aid response and in the predictability of the user of a hearing aid with specific electroacoustic performance characteristics in everyday life. However, the hearing-impaired individual requiring amplification, needs help from the hearing aid specialist now. The recommendation of a specific hearing aid must be made within the realm of scientific principles pertaining to acoustics now known and the art of hearing aid selection acquired through years of practical experience. Unfortunately, we cannot wait until the last test confirming reliability and validity of our procedures have been proven through laboratory investigation. Therefore, most specialists are involved in making hearing aid recommendations and employing one of the following methods:

SELECTIVE AMPLIFICATION

Selective amplification attempts to determine the characteristic of the hearing aid which will result in optimum performance based on the psychoacoustic information acquired through audiometric testing. There have been three schools of thought in this respect, each with its own philosophy as to the principles to be applied in arriving at the frequency-gain characteristics of the aid selected. The different theoretical approaches toward the appropriate frequency response are as follows:

1 The frequency-gain characteristic should increase in those frequency regions where the audiogram indicates that the loss is increasing in order to bring the maximum spectra of average speech at the highest sensation level into the residual auditory area without exceeding a threshold of discomfort. Most clinicians would agree with this basic principle of giving the greatest amount of gain where the individual has incurred the greatest loss. That is why most professionals recommend high-frequency emphasis in hearing aids where individuals suffer from high-frequency hearing losses (Watson and Tolan, 1949).

2 The frequency-gain characteristic resulting in optimum speech intelligibility is independent of the loss of hearing or configuration of the audiogram. This tenet was the conclusion of the Harvard Report (Davis et al., 1947) where a flat response or a response with a rise of 6dB per octave was recommended for all hearing losses (Duffy will give details as to the faulty research design of this study in chapter VII of this book). Very few clinicians would support the conclusion of the Harvard Report today, in view of the many studies reported supporting selective amplification.

3 The frequency-gain characteristic should decrease in frequency regions where the audiogram indicates the loss is greatest in order to reduce aural distortion in the ear through the stimulation of severely damaged areas of the cochlear. (Huizing and Reyntjes, 1952 and Pimonow, 1963). In fact, Pimonow proposed that the gain should be attenuated in any frequency area where the threshold level exceeds 60dB to avoid any deterioration of speech intelligibility. The only clinicians that would support this rationale would qualify the principle to limit this type of fitting to the profoundly impaired. Where a person has a profound sensorineural hearing loss with a fragmentary audiogram showing maximum hearing thresholds only in the low-frequencies and no response at maximum output of the audiometer at higher-frequencies, it has been suggested that low-frequency emphasis hearing aids be fitted to take advantage of this minimum residual hearing. The specialist must test to determine that the low-frequencies do not mask any residual hearing in the high-frequency area.

Ling (1964) stated that children with little hearing above 500Hz should receive benefit from extended low-frequency amplification. He recommended that hearing aids have a frequency range that extended down to 70Hz. However, such aids could only be worn in relatively quiet environments. Many specialists in fitting children with profound losses, still select aids which incorporate high-frequency emphasis, the degree of emphasis being dependent on the slope of the audiogram. They recommend that only for those cases where the audiogram indicated no residual hearing above 1000Hz, should the frequency range of the aid be extended as low as 100Hz.

The practitioner should be quite careful in recommending low-frequency emphasis or extended low-frequency amplification as there are cases with no response on frequencies above 1000Hz on audiometric tests but indicate high-frequency response with high gain hearing aids.

METHODS OF HEARING AID SELECTION

A. *Prescriptive Procedures*

    1 Methodology making use of formulae

        a. Based on threshold hearing levels (Berger et al., 1979; Byrne & Tonisson, 1976; Lybarger, 1978 and McCandless & Lyregaard, 1983).

        b. Based on most comfortable loudness levels, (Markle & Zaner, 1966; Victoreen, 1973 and Zelnick, 1982, 1983).

        c. Ski-slope losses (Skinner, 1976).

        d. Maximum audibility for speech spectra (Miller et al., 1980).

B. *Comparative Procedures*

    1 Speech audiometry based on following criteria (Carhart, 1946).

        a. Effective gain.

        b. Speech discrimination scores in quiet.

        c. Speech discrimination scores in noise.

        d. Tolerance.

    2 Aided sound field responses for maximum audibility.

        a. Use of pulsed or warbled pure-tones (Duffy, 1978).

        b. Use of narrow bands of noise (Pascoe, 1975).

        c. Use of damped wave trains (Victoreen, 1973).

        d. Use of amplitude modulated pure-tones (Goldberg, 1981).

    e. Use of Bekesy sweep tracings, (Fournier, 1967 and Schmitz, 1980).

3 Master hearing aid.

    a. Stationary master hearing aids.

    b. Wearable master hearing aids (Levitt & Collins, 1980).

C. *Subjective Procedures*

1 Judgments of quality of sound (Killion, 1982 and Zerlin, 1962).

2 Judgments of relative intelligibility of aided processed speech (Studebaker et al., 1980).

3 Magnitude of loudness estimation (Knight and Margolis, 1984).

D. *Objective Procedures*

1 Electroacoustic measurements in ear canal.

    a. Probe microphone (Harford, 1980).

    b. Probe tube microphone (Libby, 1985).

2 Acoustic reflex measurements (Tonisson, 1975).

3 Brain stem audiometry, unaided and aided (Jacobson et al., 1980).

E. *Combined Procedures*

Combination of any of above procedures.

A. *Current Prescriptive Formulae*

1 Lybarger Procedure (1978, method suggested in 1944).

Samuel Lybarger was among the first to support selective amplification by suggesting the one-half gain rule as a factor in hearing aid evaluation. The amplification curve was supposed to be a mirror image of approximately one-half the audiogram curve in decibels. Lybarger's suggestion was based on the premise that the hearing aid user would set the volume control of the aid to a position that would result in a preferred gain which was one-half of the air conduction threshold hearing level ($\frac{1}{2}$ of loss of hearing). Unfortunately, the one-half gain rule does not result in a presentation level for maximum speech intelligibility for all hearing-impaired users. It is my opinion, that the one-half gain rule provides too much gain for the low-frequencies and too little gain for the high-frequencies of speech, in most eases. In fairness to Sam Lybarger, I should mention the fact that

Lybarger did write that the low-frequency response should be attenuated for the most beneficial selective amplification results.

2 Berger's Procedure (1979).

This widely applied procedure will be explained and discussed in detail by Berger in chapter III of this book. To summarize, Berger suggests a fraction (close to the one-half gain rule described above) applied to the hearing threshold level in computing the frequency-gain characteristic at specific frequencies. The method also has a recommendation for SSPL at 500Hz, 1000Hz, 2000Hz and 4000Hz. The procedure also sets tolerance limits for acceptance or rejection of a specific hearing aid response by comparing the predicted gain and SSPL to real-ear measurements of gain and SSPL (sound field pure-tone testing).

3 Byrne and Tonisson Procedure (1976).

This method of hearing aid selection proposed by Byrne and Tonisson is based on the rationale that maximum speech intelligibility can be attained by having all the frequency components of speech being presented to the impaired-ear at equal loudness levels. They have derived tables that indicate the relationship between the hearing threshold level and hearing aid users' preferred gain at specific critical frequencies. This procedure used in Australia has been recently studied for its validity. Byrne & Murray (National Acoustic Laboratories of Australia) published an article in 1985 suggesting a modification of the method. Instead of using pure-tone hearing threshold levels for the selection of frequency response characteristics, they proposed the use of speech band MCLs centered at three frequencies namely, 400Hz, 1250Hz and 3150Hz. They reported that bandwidth and stimulus type both had significant effects on interfrequency differences in MCLs.

4 POGO Procedure (1983).

Prescription for gain/output for a hearing aid by McCandless and Lyregaard (1983) will be described by McCandless in chapter IV of this book. This prescriptive procedure also makes use of the one-half gain rule based on hearing threshold levels at each octave from 250Hz through 4000Hz. However, this method suggests that the gain at 250Hz be reduced by 10dB and the gain at 500Hz be reduced by 5dB. They further recommend that the predicted gain or ideal gain be verified through insertion gain measurements whereas Berger recommends verification through functional gain (sound field) measurements.

They suggest that the maximum pressure output be the average of the uncomfortable loudness levels at 500Hz, 1000Hz and 2000Hz and thus the required MPO would be expressed in dB HL. In order to convert to SPL, they add 4dB and arrive at a 2cc coupler maximum sound pressure level. POGO procedure will be explained and illustrated in detail by McCandless in chapter IV of this book. It has been applied by many specialists involved in selecting hearing aids.

5   Victoreen Procedure (1973).

Victoreen called his procedure Otometry, which he describes as both the measurement of residual hearing and its enhancement. He has suggested the use of damped-wave trains (a damped-wave train signal is a tone burst having a specified decay rate or decrement) for the determination of most comfortable loudness levels. Victoreen has proposed that the gain characteristics of the hearing aid selected bring the average amplified spectra of speech to a level which has approximately the same relationship to the threshold of audibility and the threshold of discomfort of the impaired-ear as unamplified speech presented at a comfortable level of loudness for a normal hearing ear. I have always supported Victoreen's suggestion of determining most comfortable loudness level for determining overall gain characteristic of an aid. MacAllister, a strong proponent of Otometry, will explain and describe this procedure in detail in chapter V of this book.

6   Skinner's Procedure for Ski-Slope Losses (1976).

Skinner suggested that the frequency-gain characteristic of the aid should be selected so that the levels of amplified conversational speech would fall approximately in the middle of the dynamic range of the impaired ear. The procedure stresses the concept of balance. The high-frequency emphasis required for severe high-frequency hearing loss should be restricted so that the imbalance between the low-frequency (500Hz-1000Hz) and high-frequency (2000Hz-4000Hz) presentation levels should not exceed 15dB.

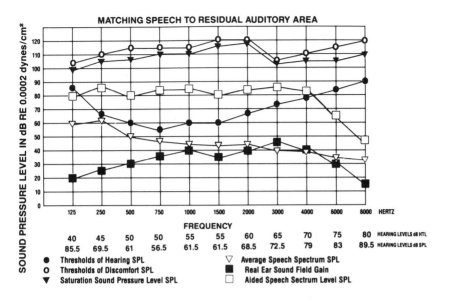

Fig. 2.

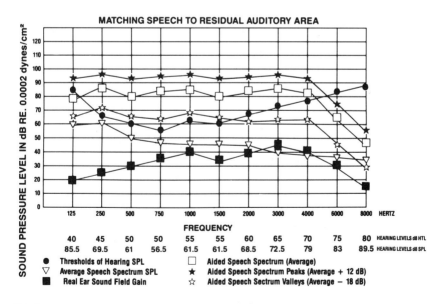

Fig. 2.

Fig. 3.

It is interesting to note that the Skinner concept of balance is in terms of the relationship of intensity of the low-frequency components of speech to the high-frequency components of speech. Whereas, Killion (1982) writes of balance in terms of frequency bandwidth. He states that research has indicated that the best tonal balance between high- and low-frequencies was obtained when the amplifier's frequency response was extended the same number of octaves above and below 800Hz. Skinner et al. (1982) reported in an article which compared speech discrimination scores for various bandwidths of a master hearing aid, the results showed the highest discrimination score for the largest bandwidth. This study would indicate that it is not necessary to cut the low-frequency response for all impaired ears indicating close to normal thresholds of hearing. Important acoustic information for vowel recognition is furnished by this frequency area. However, the intensity of the low-frequency response of the aid must be controlled so that there is no masking effect of such low-frequencies on the high-frequencies. In fact, their work would indicate that maximum speech intelligibility is attained with maximum audibility (see Figures 2 and 3 illustrating audibility for aided speech spectrum).

7 Miller et al. Procedure (1980).

Miller et al. has written on a procedure for hearing aid selection based on the audiologic description of the patient. The procedure is based on the work of Pascoe (1975) who found that there were significant differences between the sound field unaided and aided response (Pascoe called this differential functional gain) and the coupler gain (gain as determined in·a 2cc coupler). On average the coupler measurements underestimated gain at 1200 Hz by approximately 10dB and overestimated gain at 3000 Hz by approximately 20dB. Pascoe found that a frequency gain characteristic (frequency response) that truly mirrors the sound field audiogram was superior to either uniform functional gain (UFG), uniform coupler gain (UCG), a response which had a rise of 6dB per octave, or of commercial hearing aid response when tested with a master hearing aid in a signal-to-noise ratio of +6dB and a special word list loaded with difficult high-frequency phonemic distinctions.

The attempt of their procedure to mirror the sound field audiogram results in a uniform hearing level (UHL) which should give maximum audibility without exceeding the threshold of discomfort. The procedure makes use of a computer program for selection of the hearing aid with maximum performance characteristics. The client's thresholds for one-third octave bands of noise are measured unaided and aided. This measurement, properly done, reflects the gain of the hearing aid as worn by the user. It has been my experience that valid and reliable thresholds can be ascertained with the use of pulsed or warbled pure-tones in a sound field without resorting to the employment of expensive filters required for narrow noise bands.

B. *Master Hearing Aids*

1 Stationary master hearing aids.

Another approach to the selection of hearing aids by hearing aid specialists has been the use of the master hearing aid. The purpose of a master hearing aid is the convenience of changing performance characteristics such as gain, frequency response and maximum pressure output and observing which characteristics result in improved speech discrimination and quality of sound to the listener. The practitioner then selects a specific hearing aid which contains those electroacoustic characteristics which were found to give maximum benefit with the use of the master hearing aid. The specialist may also request a manufacturer to modify a particular hearing aid, in order to approximate those electroacoustic characteristics found to be desirable for a listener using a master hearing aid.

Master hearing aids are not used by many hearing aid specialists at the present time for the following reasons:

a. Many master hearing aids limited the changes that could be made in terms of gain, frequency response and maximum pressure output.

b. In many master hearing aids the specific characteristics that resulted in an appropriate fitting for a client could only be obtained from the manufacturer of the master hearing aid being employed.

c. In many cases the components used in master hearing aids are different from the actual components placed in the hearing aid ordered and the listener may complain of the changed quality of sound. Then to, the responses of the client may often differ when tested with the hearing aid assumed to have the same characteristics found appropriate when using the master hearing aid.

d. Many dispensers found that master hearing aids did not incorporate features that they desired such as, variability in compression ratios, attack and recovery times when using compression, directional and non-directional microphones and low- and high-frequency cutoffs.

e. Many master hearing aids used earphones exclusively and did not provide for the use of customized earmolds for the evaluation.

f. Currently a large percentage of hearing aids dispensed are either all-in-the-ear or all-in-the-canal types. A viable master hearing aid would have to make provision for well fitting all-in-the-ear or all-in-the-canal shells. There would still be changes in the response of the listener with the final customized hearing aid due to venting and length of the canal of the hearing aid.

g. Finally, it must be realized that with the use of a master hearing aid the signal is either introduced by speaking into a microphone in the instrument or generated within the instrument itself, whereas with a worn hearing aid the signal enters the microphone with different diffraction effects caused by the head.

2 Wearable master hearing aids.

Levitt (1978) describes a protocol for the selection of hearing aids with the use of a wearable master hearing aid. This wearable master hearing aid was specifically designed by an engineering firm for the purpose of researching the selection of hearing aids at the Graduate Center of the City University of New York. The experimental protocol being investigated by Levitt and his associates consists of four stages:

a. Baseline audiometric data.

b. Fixed experimental design.

c. Convergence phase.

d. Experimental comparisons.

A report on this study concludes that the systematic adjustment of the parameters of a wearable master hearing aid can produce improved performance and that the estimated optimum settings obtained differ significantly between subjects.

At the present time no manufacturer has produced a wearable master hearing aid. It would appear that Levitt's suggested procedure is too lengthy for practical application. Also, he has been working with a large prototype resembling a body type hearing aid and a small post-auricular or all-in-the-ear type master hearing aid is not envisioned in the immediate future.

C. *Current Objective Procedures*

1 Electroacoustic instrumentation for ear canal measurements.

a. Probe Microphone.

Harford (1980) described a procedure for the verification of the frequency response of a hearing aid while being worn by a patient through the use of miniaturized probe microphones (Starkey probe microphone system). He determined the insertion gain by measuring the unaided response at or near the eardrum as compared to the aided response with the aid at approximately the same location of the microphone in the canal. Although Harford was quite enthusiastic about this procedure for verification of insertion gain, I have not found the use of this method as feasible as others in my office practice for the following reasons:

1 Measurements often differed on re-test based on the location of the probe microphone in the external canal.

2 Ear canal into which the probe microphone is placed must be absolutely clear of all cerumen, otherwise the microphone aperture becomes occluded with debris.

3 The calibration of the miniature probe microphones is both a difficult and time consuming task.

4 The entire measuring system including probe microphones, interfacing equipment and the Phonic Ear computing instrument and test box is quite expensive.

5 The presence of the probe microphone in the ear canal causes some alteration of the frequency response.

6 Many clients whom I desired to test with a probe microphone while wearing their new hearing aid and earmold objected to the probe microphone being placed in their ear canal behind the occluded earmold (clients feared damage to their eardrums might result).

b. Probe Tube Microphone.

Recently Rastronics developed a procedure for ear canal measurements of hearing aid response without the insertion of a microphone. Instead, the procedure makes use of a tube being placed into the canal for measuring the insertion gain. The tube is connected to a microphone, external to the ear canal, which in turn feeds its output into a computerized system for gain and output measurements, usually displayed on a screen or printed. The newest type of equipment uses a computerized compression method whereby the input sound pressure level is constantly supervised and corrected by the ear. This system normally overcomes the fear of the client of having a microphone placed in the ear canal as mentioned above. In my opinion it is an excellent tool for further research on the response in the ear canal of aided acoustic stimuli. However, it must be realized that probe tube microphone measurements are electroacoustic measurements in the ear canal and are not listener behavioral responses to auditory signals. Further study is warranted to determine how well insertion gain measurements correlate with speech intelligibility and comfortability with a hearing aid. Also it must be explained how middle ear pathology or brain stem pathology affect insertion gain measured at the eardrum. The use of probe tube microphones can determine what is happening at or near the eardrum through electroacoustic data with a particular hearing aid but it does not indicate how the aid is to be modified to effectuate maximum benefit for the user. Probe microphone and probe tube microphone systems will be discussed fully in chapter VI by Preves.

SUMMARY

I have presented a history of the evolution of procedures for selection and evaluation of hearing aids over the past sixty years. The basic methodology can be classified into four categories namely; the prescriptive procedures, the comparative procedures, the subjective procedures and the objective procedures. Unfortunately, no one method has had unanimity of acceptance by professionals involved in our discipline of hearing aid selection and assessment. I have attempted to give the rationale of suggested method as described by its presenter. I have also attempted to describe the limitations of a particular methodology as I have attempted to apply the procedure in my own private practice. In addition, I have sought to present the opinions of other writers regarding their particular methods for hearing aid selection whether or not I favored them.

It appears that many practitioners are using a combined procedure for making a recommendation to a client of a particular hearing aid.

Hearing aid dispensers are using one of the prescriptive procedures for determining the performance characteristics of the aid and the subjective procedure of having the client make a final determination based on quality of sound or judgment of intelligibility. However, only real-ear measurements obtained through sound field audiometry can support the decision that an appropriate hearing aid has been selected in terms of audibility, comfortability and speech discrimination.

GLOSSARY

Bisection method A procedure of selective amplification in which the region between the threshold of hearing and the threshold of discomfort is divided in one-half and the gain of the appropriate hearing aid brings speech to this bisection level.

Coupler gain The difference between the output level of a hearing aid and the input level as measured with the use of a 2cc coupler. It is an electroacoustic measurement.

Dynamic range The dynamic range of an ear is determined by subtracting the speech reception threshold (SRT) from the threshold of discomfort (TD). It represents the range in decibels that an ear can detect and tolerate changes in sound pressure. It also applies to the range between hearing threshold (HL) and the threshold of discomfort (TD) at specific frequencies for pure-tones.

Equal loudness contours Curves which indicate the relationship that must be maintained between the sound pressure level and frequency if the pure-tones of various frequencies are to produce the same sensation of loudness. Equal-loudness contours for normal hearing listeners indicate that all pure-tones of the same sound pressure level do not sound equally as loud.

Flat response Describing a hearing aid as having a flat response means that the introduction of the amplification system does not alter the shape of the input frequency-gain characteristic. It does not mean that the output of the hearing aid will have the same intensity at all frequencies.

Frequency response The frequency response of a hearing aid is an expression of the level of amplification provided by the hearing aid for various frequencies of sound in relation to the intensity of the input signal.

Functional gain This term used by Pascoe (1975) refers to the differential between the aided threshold and the unaided threshold of hearing of a listener tested in a sound field. It is a psychoacoustic or behavioral measurement.

Gain An increase in the intensity of sound. Gain in a hearing aid is the amount in decibels by which the sound pressure level at the output from the receiver exceeds the sound pressure level introduced into the microphone.

Insertion gain The difference between the unaided sound pressure level in ear canal and the aided sound pressure level at approximately the same position in the ear canal as measured with either probe microphone or probe tube microphone. It is an electroacoustic measurement.

Mirroring the audiogram This procedure of selecting a hearing aid by providing sufficient gain to compensate for the loss of hearing shown by the audiogram. The new concept of mirroring attempts to mirror the audiogram in shaping the frequency response of the hearing aid and not in terms of absolute gain.

Most comfortable loudness level (MCL) The sound pressure level at which the listener finds the intensity of the acoustic signal most pleasant or comfortable.

Otometry The term first used by Victoreen (1973) refers to the science dealing with sensation of loudness created by sound pressures. It is concerned with the selection of electroacoustic characteristics of hearing aids based on the determination of most comfortable loudness sound pressures.

Phonemic scoring A method of partial-scoring of correctly recognized phonemes as a means of determining speech discrimination scores, suggested by Duffy (1967).

POGO A procedure for determining the gain and output characteristics of hearing aids based on the one-half gain rule as proposed by McCandless and Lyregaard (1983).

Probe microphone A miniaturized microphone for measuring sound pressure generated by a hearing aid within the ear canal.

Real-ear response The measurement of unaided thresholds and aided thresholds in a sound field using various acoustic signals such as pulsed or warbled pure-tones, narrow bands of noise, damped wave trains and amplitude modulated pure-tones. It is a psychoacoustic or behavioral measurement and has often been referred to as functional gain.

Saturation Sound Pressure Level The greatest sound intensity an amplifying system can produce. SSPL 90 curve refers to output of hearing aid with an input signal of 90dB SPL and gain control in full on position.

Selective amplification A philosophy of selecting hearing aid characteristics of gain, frequency response and maximum pressure output are based on the audiometric profile of the hearing impaired individual. There are many procedures proposed for selective amplification, some based on most comfortable loudness and others based on the threshold audiogram.

Sensation level The sensation level of a sound is the number of decibels by which the intensity level of the sound exceeds the absolute threshold of a particular ear for that sound.

Signal-to-noise ratio The ratio of the intensity of an acoustic signal to the intensity of the residual noise in the absence of the acoustic signal. Example, if the speech signal is 65dB and the background noise is 60dB, the signal-to-noise ratio would be +5dB.

Sound field A room or particular area in which the acoustic signals originate from loudspeakers. The room is usually constructed with surfaces of sound absorbent material to avoid the occurrence of standing waves.

Sound pressure level (SPL) Sound pressure level, stated in decibels, is a logarithmic ratio of the measured sound pressure and a reference sound pressure (.0002 dynes per cm/^{2}).

Speech discrimination scores (SDS) A score resulting from a test of the ability to understand speech as determined by scoring the number of words in a phonetically balanced list repeated correctly.

Speech spectrum The relationship of the intensity level of speech to frequency. The average conversational level of speech is approximately 65dB SPL. The dynamic range of average speech is 28dB (Fletcher, 1926). The frequency range for good speech intelligibility is from 200Hz-8000Hz, although the frequency range for audibility of a normal ear is from 20Hz-20,000Hz.

Suprathreshold Acoustic stimuli presented above the threshold of hearing.

Threshold of discomfort (TD) The sound pressure level or the intensity of an acoustic signal which will produce a sensation of discomfort or annoyance. In a normal ear it is usually about 120dB SPL, however, it can be lower in a sensorineural hearing-impaired ear.

Threshold of hearing The minimum level of intensity of an acoustic stimulus which can be heard correctly 50% of the time. When measured with an audiometer, it is recorded as HL or HTL referenced by the calibration of the audiometer in either ANSI or ISO.

Uniform hearing level The uniform hearing level is the basis of a method which selects the electroacoustic performance characteristics, and frequency-gain, based on mirroring the soundfield audiogram. (Pascoe, 1975). The soundfield audiogram is mirrored in terms of shape but not absolutely in terms of gain.

REFERENCES

BERGER, K. W., HAGBERG, E. N. & RANE, R. L. (1979): "Prescription of Hearing Aids: Rationale, Procedure, and Results", Revised edition, Herald Publishing House, Kent, Ohio.

BYRNE, D. & TONISSON, W. (1976): "Selecting the gain of hearing aids for persons with sensorineural hearing impairments". *Scand. Audiology*, 5, pp. 51-59.

BYRNE, D. & MURRAY, N. (1985): "Relationships of HTLs, MCLs, LDLs and psychoacoustic tuning curves to the optimal frequency response characteristics of hearing aids". *The Australian Journal of Audiology*, Vol. 7, No. 1, pp. 7-16.

CARHART, R. (1946): "Tests for the selection of hearing aids". *Laryngoscope*, 56, pp. 780-794.

CARHART, R. (1950): "Hearing aid selection by university clinics". *Journal of Speech and Hearing Disorders*, 15, pp. 106-113.

DAVIS, H., STEVENS, S. S., NICHOLS, R. H., JR., HUDGINS, C. V., MARQUIS, R. J., PETERSON, G. E. and ROSS, D. A. (1947): "Hearing Aids, An Experimental Study of Design Objectives, Harvard University Press, Cambridge, Mass.

DUFFY, J. K. (1967): "Audio-visual speech audiometry and a new audio and audio-visual speech perception index". *Maico Audiological Library Series*, Vol. V, Report 9, pp. 1-3.

DUFFY, J. K. (1978): "Sound field audiometry and hearing aid advisements". *Hearing Instruments*, Vol. 29, No. 2, pp. 6-12.

DUFFY, J. K. & ZELNICK, E. (1985): "A critique of past and current hearing aid assessment procedures". *Audecibel*, Fall, pp. 10-23.

DUGAL, R. L., BRAIDA, L. D. & DURLACH, N. I. (1980): "Implications of previous research for the selection of frequency-gain characteristics". In G. A. Studebaker and I. Hochberg (Eds.) Acoustical Factors Affecting Hearing Aid Performance, University Park Press, Baltimore, Md., pp. 379-403.

FLETCHER, H. (1926): "Hopeful trends in the testing of hearing aids and in the prescription of hearing aids". Paper given before the 50th annual meeting of the American Federation of Organizations for the Hard of Hearing.

FOURNIER, J. E. (1968): "Hearing aid evaluation by pure tone automatic audiometry". *Audecibel*, 17, pp. 99-108.

GOLDBERG, H. (1981): "Sound field audiometric measurements". *Audecibel*, 30, pp. 183-186.

HARFORD, E. R. (1980): "The use of a miniature microphone in the ear canal for the verification of hearing aid performance". *Ear and Hearing*, Vol. 1, No. 6, pp. 329-337.

HUIZING, H. C., & REYNTJES, J. A. (1952): "Recruitment and speech discrimination loss". *Laryngoscope*, 62 pp. 521-527.

JACOBSON, J. T., SEITZ, M. R., MENCHER, G. T., and PARROTT, V. (1980): "Auditory brainstem response: a contribution to infant assessment and management". In G. T. Mencher and S. E. Gerber, (Eds.), *Early Management of Hearing Loss*, New York: Grune and Stratton, pp. 151-181.

KILLION, M. C. (1982): "Transducers, earmolds and sound quality considerations". In G. A. Studebaker and F. H. Bess, (Eds.), *The Vanderbilt Hearing-Aid Report*, Monographs in Contemporary Audiology, Darby, Pa., pp. 109-110.

KNIGHT, K. K., MARGOLIS, R. H. (1984): "Magnitude estimation of loudness: loudness perception in presbycusic listeners". *Journal of Speech and Hearing Research*, Vol. 27, No. 1, pp. 28-32.

KNUDSEN, V. & JONES, I. (1936): "Audiometry and the prescribing of hearing aid". *Laryngoscope*, 46, pp. 523-536.

LEVITT, H. & COLLINS, M. J. (1980): "An experimental protocol for the prescriptive fitting of a wearable master hearing aid". In G. A. Studebaker and I. Hochberg (Eds.), Acoustical Factors Affecting Hearing Aid Performance, University Park Press, Baltimore, Md., pp. 323-339.

LIBBY, E. R. (1985): "State-of-the-art of hearing aid selection procedures". *Hearing Instruments*, Vol. 36, No. 1 pp. 30-36.

LING, D. (1964): "Implications of hearing aid amplification below 300 cps". *Volta Review*, 66, pp. 723-729.

LYBARGER, S. F. (1978): "Selective amplification — a review and evaluation". *Journal of the American Audiology Society*, the Williams & Wilkins Co. Vol. 3, No. 6, pp. 259-260. (Patent Application S.N. 543, 278 vy S. F. Lybarger, 7/1944).

MARKLE, D. M. & ZANER, A. (1966): "The determination of 'gain requirements' of hearing aids: a new method". *The Journal of Auditory Research*, Vol. 6, No. 4, pp. 371-377.

McCANDLESS, G. A. & LYREGAARD, P. E. (1983): "Prescription of gain/output (POGO) for hearing aids". *Hearing Instruments*, Vol. 34, No. 1, pp. 16-21.

MILLER, J. D., NIEMOELLER, A. F., PASCOE, D. & SKINNER, M. W. (1980): "Integration of the electroacoustic description of hearing aids with the audiologic description of clients". In G. A. Studebaker and I. Hochberg (Eds.), Acoustical Factors Affecting Hearing Aid Performance, University Park Press, Baltimore, Md., pp. 355-377.

MILLIN, J. P. (1980): "Practical and philosophical considerations". In M. C. Pollack, Amplification for the Hearing-Impaired (second edition), Grune and Stratton, Inc. New York, N.Y., pp. 143-176.

OLSEN, W. & WILBER, S. (1967): "Physical performance characteristics of different hearing aids and speech discrimination scores achieved with them by hearing-impaired persons". Paper given before the American Speech and Hearing Association, Chicago, Ill.

PASCOE, D. P. (1975): "Frequency responses of hearing aids and their effects on the speech perception of hearing-impaired subjects". *Annals of Otology, Rhinology and Laryngology*, 84, supplement 23.

PETERSON, G. E. & LEHISTE, I. (1962): "Revised CNC lists for auditory tests". *Journal of Speech and Hearing Disorders*, 27, pp. 62-70.

PIMONOW, L. (1963): "The application of synthetic speech to aural rehabilitation". *Journal of Auditory Research*, 3, pp. 73-82.

RAFFIN, M. J. M., & THORTON, A. R. (1980): "Confidence levels for differences between speech-discrimination scores". *Journal of Speech and Hearing Research*, 23, pp. 5-18.

RESNICK, D. & BECKER, M. (1963): "Hearing aid evaluation — a new approach", *American Speech and Hearing Association Journal*, 5, pp. 695-699.

SCHARF, B. & FLORENTINE, M. (1982): "Psychoacoustics of elementary sounds". In G. A. Studebaker and Fred H. Bess, (Eds.) *The Vanderbilt Hearing-Aid Report*, Monographs in Contemporary Audiology, Darby, Pa., pp. 3-15.

SCHMITZ, H. D. (1980): "Hearing aid selection for adults". In M. C. Pollack, Amplification for the Hearing-Impaired (second edition), Grune & Stratton, Inc. New York, N.Y., pp. 177-211.

SCHWARTZ, D. M. & WALDEN, B. E. (1980): "Current status of the clinical hearing aid evaluation". In Studies In The Use of Amplification for the Hearing Impaired. Excerpta Medica, pp. 15-28.

SCHWARTZ, D. M. & WALDEN, B. E. (1983): "Speech audiometry and hearing aid assessment". In D. F. Konkle and W. R. Rintlemann, (Eds.), Principles of Speech Audiometry, University Park Press, Baltimore, Md., pp. 321-352.

SHORE, I., BILGER, R. C. & HIRSH, I. J. (1960): "Hearing aid evaluation: reliability of repeated measurements". *Journal of Speech and Hearing Research*, 25, pp. 152-170.

SKINNER, M. W. (1976): "Speech intelligibility in noise-induced hearing loss: effects of high-frequency compensation". Unpublished Ph.D. thesis, Washington University, St. Louis, Mo.

SKINNER, M. W., PASCOE, D. P., MILLER, J. D. & POPELKA, G. R. (1982): "Measurements to determine the optimal placement of speech energy within the listener's auditory area: a basis for selecting amplification characteristics". In G. A. Studebaker and F. H. Bess, (Eds.) *The Vanderbilt Hearing-Aid Report*, Monographs in Contemporary Audiology, Darby, Pa., pp. 161-169.

STUDEBAKER, G. A. (1980): "Hearing aid selection: an overview". In G. A. Studebaker and F. H. Bess, (Eds.) *The Vanderbilt Hearing-Aid Report*, Monographs in Contemporary Audiology, Darby, Pa., pp. 147-155.

TONISSON, W. (1975): "Measuring in-the-ear gain of hearing aid by acoustic reflex method". *Journal of Speech and Hearing Research*, 18, pp. 17-30.

VICTOREEN, J. A. (1973): Basic Principles of Otometry. Charles C. Thomas, Springfield, Ill.

WALLENFELS, H. G. (1967): Hearing Aids on Prescription. Charles C. Thomas, Springfield, Ill.

WATSON, N. A. & KNUDSON, V. D. (1940): "Selective amplification in hearing aids". *Journal of Acoustical Society of America*, 11, pp. 406-419.

WATSON, N. A. & TOLAN, T. (1949): Hearing Tests and Hearing Instruments. Williams and Wilkins, Baltimore, Md.

WEST, R., KENNEDY, L. & CARR, A. (1937): The Rehabilitation of Speech. Harper and Brothers, New York, N.Y., p. 9.

ZELNICK, E. (1970): "Comparison of speech perception utilizing monotic and dichotic modes of listening". *Journal of Auditory Research*, 10, pp. 87-97.

ZELNICK, E. (1982): "Selecting frequency response". *Hearing Aid Journal*. Vol. 35, No. 3, March issue, p. 31.

ZELNICK, E. (1982): "A comparison of procedures for hearing aid evaluation". *Audecibel*, Part I, Fall 1982, pp. 32-38.

ZELNICK, E. (1983): "A comparison of procedures for hearing aid evaluation". *Audecibel*, Part II, Winter 1983, pp. 21-26.

ZERLIN, S. (1962): "A new approach to hearing aid selection". *Journal of Speech and Hearing Research*, 5, pp. 370-376.

II

MODES OF AMPLIFICATION

ERNEST ZELNICK

INTRODUCTION

The person evaluated for a hearing aid must be tested audiometrically. When the audiometric data indicates that the individual is a candidate for a hearing aid, medical clearance in conformance with the Food and Drug Administration regulations should be secured. The decision must now be made by the hearing aid specialist as to which mode of amplification would be most appropriate in fitting the client's hearing loss.

Manufacturers of hearing aids have made five modes of amplification commercially available for fitting hearing impairments. The modes of amplification currently available are: monaural, binaural, bilateral (Y-cord), CROS and BICROS.

Research over the years on modes of amplification has furnished to those specializing in hearing aid selection, rationale for the preference of one mode over another for specific hearing losses. It is true that many individuals are fitted monaurally because both the public and the specialist involved in dispensing have the attitude that most people can be helped appreciably by amplification to one ear. A recent article indicates that the attitude of both the dispenser and the recipient of the aid is quite important as to the decision as to which mode will be selected.

I have written extensively supporting binaural hearing aid fittings. Many psychoacoustic principles are discussed in this chapter demonstrating the importance of two-eared fittings if the bilaterally hearing-impaired are to have speech perception restored to normal or near normal function through amplification. It is not to be assumed that every individual with a bilateral hearing loss is a suitable candidate for binaural fittings, examples are described where the practitioner must test carefully to avoid a degradation effect by providing amplification to the second ear.

There are individuals suffering from a unilateral hearing loss who cannot be aided with a monaural fitting. For these cases CROS and BICROS systems of amplification will be illustrated and their benefits discussed.

In the case where a monaural fitting is the appropriate means of amplification or where the client refuses to accept binaural hearing aids, the decision of which ear to fit becomes critical. I have listed and discussed rules for monaural hearing aid fittings. The use of the guidelines enumerated for maximum benefit from a monaural fitting have resulted in acceptance of the hearing aid by many individuals that I have fitted.

CHAPTER OBJECTIVES

The primary purpose of this chapter is to acquaint the reader with the various modes of amplification available in commercial hearing aids. Binaural hearing aid fittings have gained greater acceptability by both the professional involved in hearing aid selection and by the hearing-impaired. This chapter attempts to acquaint dispensers of hearing aids with the many advantages of binaural hearing.

This chapter provides a rationale for the ear to be selected for monaural amplification. The hearing aid specialist will find many of the rules listed for selecting the ear to be aided quite helpful in his daily practice.

In addition the diotic mode (Y-cord) is explained and its limited use for young children discussed.

Special fittings for the unilateral hearing-impaired are presented through the explanation of the CROS and BICROS modes of amplification. The reader should become better acquainted with the various modifications of CROS hearing aids to better fit his particular client.

Bone conduction oscillators and amplification systems are still being designed and the author hopes to acquaint hearing aid dispensers with their use when required.

MODES OF AMPLIFICATION

There are actually five modes of amplification available for hearing aid fittings that manufacturers are producing. I will describe the various modes of amplification suggesting the advantages accruing from their application. Since I feel that the specialist in selecting appropriate amplification for the hearing-impaired should attempt to achieve maximum speech intelligibility, I have started the description of amplifying modes with binaural hearing aids, the mode most likely to result in optimum hearing benefits.

A. Binaural mode of amplification contains two independent channels; a separate microphone, a separate receiver and a separate amplifier. Each channel delivers the amplified acoustic output to one ear (see Figure 1).

B. Monaural mode of amplification contains one microphone, one receiver and one amplifier. The amplified acoustic output is delivered to either the better or poorer ear (see Figure 2).

C. Diotic (Y-cord arrangement) mode of amplification contains one microphone, two receivers and one amplifier. The acoustic output is delivered through the Y-cord to both ears (see Figure 3).

D. CROS (contralateral routing of signal) mode of amplification contains one microphone, one receiver and one amplifier. The microphone is placed either in an eyeglass temple, a post-auricular shell or an all-in-the ear shell and the amplifier and receiver are placed in a contralaterally worn eyeglass temple or shell enabling acoustic signals

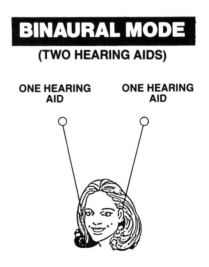

BINAURAL MODE
(TWO HEARING AIDS)

ONE HEARING AID   ONE HEARING AID

Fig. 1.

MONAURAL MODE

**TO BETTER EAR
ONE HEARING AID**

**TO POORER EAR
ONE HEARING AID**

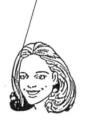

Fig. 2.

DIOTIC MODE (Y-CORD) TO BOTH EARS

**Y-CORD
IN PARALLEL
IMPEDANCE
TO MATCH
AID (Z)**

**OUTPUT OF ONE
HEARING AID FED
TO TWO RECEIVERS**

**Y-CORD
IN SERIES
IMPEDANCE
TO MATCH
AID (Z)**

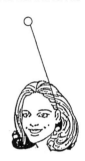

**IMPEDANCE
OF EACH
RECEIVER
(2XZ)**

**IMPEDANCE
OF EACH
RECEIVER
(1/2 Z)**

Fig. 3.

received on one side of the head to be delivered amplified to the contralateral ear.

E. BICROS mode of amplification contains two microphones (one microphone placed in a post auricular shell, eyeglass temple or all-in-ear shell and the second microphone placed in a contralateral post auricular shell, eyeglass temple or all-in-ear shell), one receiver and one amplifier. The BICROS can be used with either an open or occluding mold dependent on the severity of the loss in the better ear.

A. *Binaural Mode of Amplification*

A logical goal of any hearing aid selection methodology is to select electroacoustic amplification that would achieve normal, or as near normal hearing response as possible for a specific hearing loss. Since normal hearing people achieve normal listening responses through the use of two ears, it would seem sensible to assume that the hearing-impaired individuals would require the use of their two ears for maximum listening benefit.

For over twenty-five years, in my articles and lectures, I have been an ardent advocate of binaural hearing aid fittings. I have suggested that binaural hearing aids be strongly recommended by professionals engaged in hearing aid evaluation, whenever the audiometric data indicates such need on the part of their client.

When an individual suffering from a bilateral loss of hearing is fitted with a monaural hearing aid, such a person cannot be expected to hear normally, as he or she will still suffer from a unilateral hearing loss even though maximum response is achieved by amplification to the aided ear. It must be realized that appropriate amplification alone does not always result in normal speech intelligibility, as most people with sensorineural hearing losses have problems in frequency selectivity (the ability to select among simultaneous presented frequencies), temporal resolution (ability to separate auditory events in respect to time) in addition to the reduced sensitivity (hearing threshold) of the ear for acoustic signals. The hearing aid essentially attempts to make speech louder (more intense) in those frequency areas where a hearing loss exists.

The hearing aid specialist in order to accomplish an appropriate fitting must make every effort to provide audibility for speech in both ears through amplification. The widest bandwidth of the speech spectrum should be amplified into the residual auditory area in both ears in order to maximize speech discrimination.

Historically, most opponents of binaural hearing aid fittings have argued that there has been a failure to demonstrate clinically the benefits of binaural amplification. Not only has the results of many satisfied binaural hearing aid users justified my recommendations, but I have also cited a number of laboratory and clinical studies demonstrating the advantages accruing from binaural hearing and binaural amplification. Some of the psychoacoustic advantages of binaural hearing aid fittings are:

1 *Localization*

Most normal hearing persons can localize the source of sound in the median plane to an accuracy of approximately one degree. They can also judge the distance of sources of sound, as well as the angle of elevation. When multiple sounds arrive at the ears simultaneously from different sources, the listener using both ears is able to selectively sort them out and locate their specific sources. Although, this process of auditory localization can be often accomplished with only one functioning ear (by rapid head movements), such monaural localization has proven to be much less accurate than when both ears are used. Localization of sound sources is dependent on interaural differences in intensity, time, phase and spectra (frequency). For people with bilateral hearing losses, the only way to achieve interaural differences is through binaural amplification (Zelnick, 1980). Again, there are skeptics who have argued that localization effects are not possible with the use of hearing aids. A recent study by Westermann and Topholm (1985) concluded that the use of two ITEs (In-The-Ear hearing aids) increased directional hearing appreciably. The subjects of their study were able to localize sound sources more accurately with binaural all-in-the-ear aids than without hearing aids or with the use of binaural postauricular amplification.

2 *Improved Speech Discrimination in Noise*

Most research on binaural hearing has indicated that the true advantage of two-eared hearing is elicited under poor listening conditions. In fact, I wrote (Zelnick, 1970):

> "if the benefits of binaural hearing are to be demonstrated, speech stimuli and competing noise would have to be presented at such relative intensities so that the relationship between the two results in a masking effect which prevents one ear from functioning as well as both ears."

Broadbent (1956) has suggested that the ability to listen to one signal, usually speech, while disregarding a signal, is increased through the use of two ears. Foreground and background relationships can be crystalized much more effectively when three dimensionality is preserved in the auditory environment through binaural hearing.

There are those in our discipline who would argue that better speech intelligibility in a background of noise through the use of binaural hearing only applies to the normal hearing population. However, Harris (1965) and Zelnick (1970) have reported in separate studies that listeners with bilateral hearing-impairments showed significant improvement in speech discrimination when using the binaural mode of amplification. In fact, I found that when scoring speech discrimination with the phonemic method as suggested by Duffy (1967), a much more sensitive measure of speech recognition than the conventional all-or-nothing method, that the binaural system of listening proved significantly superior for speech intelligibility to the monaural mode. Markides (1977) also concluded that individuals with symmetrical as well as asymmetrical hearing-impairments showed binaural advantages for speech perception when utilizing amplification in both ears. Most professionals in our discipline are convinced that there is sufficient evidence that binaural hearing improves speech intelligibility, not only in quiet but especially in difficult (noisy) listening situations.

3   *Head-Shadow Effect*

Probably, the most effective argument for the recommendation and fitting of binaural hearing aids is the head-shadow effect. The interposition of the head to a source of sound produces interaural intensive disparities especially affecting the high-frequency components of speech. Low-frequency tones, having longer wave-lengths, are better able to be routed around the barrier of the head to the contralateral ear and are therefore heard at a higher intensity (increased loudness) than the high-frequency tones. The high-frequency components of speech, having shorter wave-lengths, are not diffracted around the head and therefore their intensities are attenuated to a much greater degree than low-frequency sounds. This disparity in intensity between the near ear and the contralateral or far ear results in significant differences in the signal-to-noise ratios at each ear. (The actual signal-to-noise ratio at a particular ear depends on the intensity and angle of incidence of the source of speech and the intensity and the angle of incidence to the particular ear of the source of noise.) Tillman et al. (1963) found a 6.4dB difference in the spondee threshold source when such source was at a 45° azimuth from the center of the head. Depending on the source of speech and the source of noise, the signal-to-noise ratios at each ear will vary and the difference between two effective signal-to-noise ratios at each ear can be as much as 13dB; resulting in a large masking effect at the ear which has a greater intensity of noise than of speech (Figure 4). The intensity of speech will be much greater than the intensity of noise at the ear contralateral to the source of noise. Since such head-shadow effects occur constantly in everyday listening situations, a binaural listener has a tremendous advantage over the person hearing with only one ear. The two-eared listener can take advantage of a particular situation and favor the ear contralateral to the source of noise and thus having the better signal-to-noise ratio. The normal hearing listener or the listener wearing two hearing aids can position himself so that one ear is toward the source of the desired speech. Whereas, the person with unilateral hearing or wearing one hearing aid and having his normal or aided ear toward the source of noise will be unable to effectively discriminate speech in the background of noise.

4 *Summation Effect*

The binaural summation effect at threshold is approximately 3dB. However, no one desires to hear at threshold; in fact most studies have indicated maximum speech intelligibility is achieved at a sensation level 30dB to 40dB above

Head Shadow Effect Using Two Loudspeakers In Sound Field

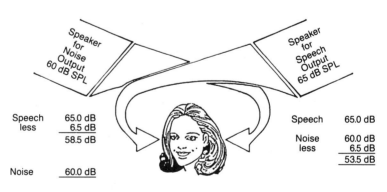

Fig. 4. Attenuation of 6.5 dB due to diffraction effect by head.

threshold. Causse and Chavasse (1942) reported that at binaural sensation level of 35dB, equal-loudness was obtained with a monaural listening condition, with a 6dB differential in the intensity of the sound. This supra-threshold summation effect enables individuals to receive sufficient gain from binaurally worn ear-level hearing aids even though they may have severe losses of hearing and would need greater gain with monaural use. In many cases, such individuals cannot achieve comfortable loudness when wearing monaural hearing aids. Therefore, many clinicians have been recommending high-gain ear-level binaural hearing aid fittings for children with severe and profound hearing losses, thus taking advantage of the supra-threshold summation effect to effectuate the desired comfortable loudness levels.

5 Sensory Deprivation

There appears to be evidence that binaural auditory sensory deprivation can effect binaural function. Beggs and Foreman (1980) reported that the critical period for binaural stimulation occurs between the ages of four and eight years. It, therefore, becomes critical that binaural hearing aids be fitted as early as possible following the conclusion that a child has a bilateral hearing loss, to avoid sensory deprivation.

The question of the effects of auditory deprivation in adults suffering from bilateral sensorineural hearing loss has only recently been investigated. Silman, Gelfand and Silverman, (1980) conducted a study at the Veterans Administration Medical Center in New Jersey with 44 adults suffering from bilateral sensorineural hearing loss who were fitted with monaural hearing aids, and 23 adult males with bilateral sensorineural hearing loss who were fitted with binaural hearing aids. Their performance based on pure-tone and speech audiometric tests conducted prior to the use of hearing aids was compared to their performance after four to five years of hearing aid use. The results of the comparison revealed that the speech recognition scores of the binaurally fitted subjects remained stable over time, whereas there were significant differences over time with the monaural hearing aid group for their unaided ears. The diminishment in speech discrimination in the unaided ears appears to be the result of auditory deprivation over the four to five year period. It therefore becomes the responsibility of the professionals involved in hearing aid selection to recommend binaural hearing aids whenever the audiometric profile indicates such need.

I would be interested to learn whether or not the diminishment of speech discrimination in the unfitted ears of the group having bilateral hearing losses and wearing monaural hearing aids would be reversible through the introduction of amplification by binaural hearing aid fitting.

6 *Quality of Sound*

Many current writers on hearing aid evaluation are suggesting that the quality of the sound from the aid is an important factor influencing the acceptance of amplification by the hearing-impaired. In fact, many of us who have been involved in hearing aid selection for many years have suggested a multi-dimensional approach of using both warbled tones and speech soundfield audiometry as well as qualitative judgments by the users in selecting hearing aids.

Killion (1982) suggested that the main reason so many users accepted binaural hearing aids, even though there was a failure to demonstrate increased speech intelligibility by the use of the second aid, was simply that the sound quality with two hearing aids was much better than with one. It has also been my experience that many new users readily accept binaural hearing aid fittings whereas there is a much more difficult adjustment to a monaural hearing aid. It appears to me that based on users' response, the quality of sound is better with binaural fittings.

I have explained in Chapter I, that although qualitative judgments are important in hearing aid selections, it should be the basis of a final selection only after sound field testing and speech audiometry (using phonemic scoring) has indicated that particular aids are furnishing appropriate gain and frequency response for the hearing-impaired ear (see Duffy chapter VII).

7 *Ease of Listening*

Almost thirty years ago Bergman (1957) reported in a study on hearing-impaired blind people, that many of his subjects commented that they had experienced a greater ease of listening when hearing with both ears or binaural hearing aids rather than with one ear or one hearing aid.

It has also been my observation that many hearing-impaired persons are more relaxed and under less tension in a listening situation when using the binaural mode of amplification rather than the monaural mode. This observation has been verified by parents and educators of children with bilateral hearing impairments, as well as by the thousands of adults wearing hearing aids in both ears.

8 *Capacity of the Auditory System*

Any listener has a limited capacity for handling information presented auditorily. The advantage of binaural hearing will manifest itself normally under poor listening conditions. It is only when there are sounds which are interfering with the speech message and the monaural listener cannot function at his maximum information handling capacity, that the value of the second ear becomes evident. It is the additional auditory cues furnished by the second ear that enable the listener to better perceive speech. The dichotic (binaural) mode of listening does not increase the individual's capacity for handling information, but it does maximize the ability to reach this capacity when acoustic conditions exist that interfere with the ability of one ear to function at its maximum.

9 *Squelch Effect*

The ability of the auditory system to suppress disturbing sounds in the environment has been described as the squelch effect. Investigators have reported that listening under earphones to reproductions of a reverberant environment was much more disturbing when presented either monaurally or diotically (Y-cord) rather than binaurally. The binaural reception, when separate microphones were used for each earphone, resulted in a disturbing sound fading in loudness and becoming more tolerable to the listener (Koenig, 1950). It appears that the binaural listener is able to selectively attend to any particular signal and disregard the background of complex sounds. It has been found that the acoustic squelch effect can enable the dichotic signal to be increased by an additional 12dB without becoming annoying or objectionable to the listener. It is evident that listening under earphones creates a condition which is similar to that of a hearing aid user and similar auditory perceptions should be experienced. Therefore, binaural hearing aids should enhance the selectivity of auditory signals and suppress interfering background noise.

10 *Binaural Masking Level Differences (BMLD)*

Licklider (1948) reported his observations on speech intelligibility when masking speech by white noise. His measurements on the intelligibility of speech presented dichotically (binaurally) under each of six interaural phase relations (see Table 1), used fixed levels of intensity of speech and of noise. The speech and noise can be in phase or out of phase at the eardrum of each ear. Licklider classified the phasic relationships as antiphasic (speech in phase and noise out of phase or noise in phase and speech out of phase), homophasic (speech in phase and noise in phase or speech out of phase and noise out of phase) and heterophasic (speech in phase and noise randomized in phase at each ear or speech out of phase and noise randomized at each ear). His report indicated speech discrimination scores were the highest when speech was out of phase and noise was in phase between the two ears (antiphasic, see Table 2).

Licklider further reported that the interaural phase effect was greater at low speech-to-noise ratios than at higher speech-to-noise ratios. It appears, that the interaural phase effects on speech intelligibility are elicited better under poor listening conditions. Although recent research indicates that the binaural masking level differences are not as large for sensorineural hearing-impaired as for listeners with normal hearing, they still show better speech intelligibility for the antiphasic condition of dichotic (binaural) listening.

Manufacturers of hearing aids have attempted to take advantage of the binaural masking level difference to enhance speech discrimination. Johnson (1975) describes a binaural hearing instrument, the BiPhasic hearing aid (Zenith), in which a phase difference is introduced between the two amplifiers of a binaural eyeglass hearing aid. Briskey (1972) reported that when supplying a person with binaural hearing aids that are 180° out of phase with each other, the individual experienced a greater capacity for processing the binaural information and accepted the use of amplification more readily.

It is very difficult to create an antiphasic relationship between the two amplifiers of a binaural hearing aid as the reversal of phase causes both the noise and speech to be out of phase between the ears. To accomplish the antiphasic condition it is necessary to change the phase of either

INTERAURAL PHASE RELATIONS

ORDER OF INTELLIGIBILITY	SPEECH	NOISE	SYMBOL	CLASS
1	OUT OF PHASE	IN PHASE	– +	ANTIPHASIC
2	IN PHASE	OUT OF PHASE	+ –	ANTIPHASIC
3	IN PHASE	RANDON PHASE	+ 0	HETEROPHASIC
4	OUT OF PHASE	RANDOM PHASE	– 0	HETEROPHASIC
5	IN PHASE	IN PHASE	+ +	HOMOPHASIC
6	OUT OF PHASE	OUT OF PHASE	– –	HOMOPHASIC

Table 1. Possible phase relationships: + in phase, – out of phase, 0 random phase.

MONAURAL-BINAURAL PRESENTATION AND INTERAURAL PHASE RELATIONS AS FACTORS INFLUENCING THE MASKING OF SPEECH BY WHITE NOISE.

SPEECH	NOISE				
	BINAURAL			MONAURAL	
	+	0	–	R	L
BINAURAL +	18.0	27.4	35.4	98.0	99.0
BINAURAL –	43.0	27.3	15.8	98.1	98.8
MONAURAL R	30.3	13.2	20.1	16.6	98.7
MONAURAL L	18.1	8.3	15.2	98.4	15.4

Table 2. Mean speech discrimination scores under various phase relationships reported by Licklider: + in phase, – out of phase, 0 random phase, R right ear, and L left ear.

speech or the noise in one ear compared to the other. This intra-aural change of phase of components amplified to one ear can be achieved electronically in the laboratory as was done by Licklider, but cannot be easily produced in a wearable binaural hearing aid.

11 *Adaptation to Hearing Aids by Geriatrics*

There is very often a period of adjustment and adaptation when a person is fitted with a hearing aid for the first time and even when a user purchases a new hearing aid. The individual must learn to recognize and understand the phonemes of speech that in some cases have never been heard (deafness existing at birth or arising in early infancy) and in other cases that he may not have heard for many years (presbycusis). The longer a person has suffered from a hearing loss without having the benefit of amplification, the more difficult it is for the recognition mechanism in the auditory central pathway to adapt to the new speech code being received through the use of a hearing aid.

When a client is first fitted with a hearing aid, there most likely will exist a mismatch between the acoustic code of the input to the recognition device and the performance of such device in the auditory system. Such mismatch will gradually decrease as the client uses the hearing aid, as a result of adaptation on the part of the hearing-impaired individual (Barford, 1979). It, therefore, has appeared logical to me that since the learned patterns of decoding of acoustic signals into understandable speech has been learned by using two ears, binaural amplification should make the adaptation process much easier and shorter for the average presbyacusic client.

12 *Tinnitus*

Most investigations and reports on effective methods of masking tinnitus (internal noise in the ear or in the head) have indicated that the best masking device has been the use of a hearing aid. Since many tinnitus sufferers have bilateral hearing losses as well as tinnitus in both ears, binaural hearing aids should be recommended as the monaural hearing aid will only alleviate the noise in one ear but will have the client complaining of tinnitus in the other ear.

13 *Effects of Reverberation Reduced by Binaural Hearing Aid Fittings*

Hearing-impaired individuals are affected by either noise or reverberation to a greater extent than normal hearing persons. Masking of the speech signal is increased by adding reverberation to ambient noise. Nabelek (1982) conducted a study of speech perception in noise and reverberation with hearing-impaired subjects. The conclusion of this study was that hearing-impaired listeners indicated an advantage for speech intelligibility when listening binaurally compared to the monaural condition. The significant advantage indicated for binaural hearing over the monotic mode was maintained with the introduction of hearing aids. This is another illustration of binaural advantages also being evident with binaural amplification.

Nabelek and Pickett (1974) reported better speech discrimination scores with the binaural over the monaural mode of listening for both normal and hearing-impaired listeners in backgrounds of noise at different reverberation times.

14 *Integration or Fusion Effect*

Integration is defined as the central auditory mechanism for the unification or fusion of auditory signals from both ears into a unitary image. Whenever dissimilar reproduction of the same speech sample are heard binaurally, integration can occur. Integration results in the acoustic signal presented at the two ears being perceived as one fused image. Furthermore, the integration of incomplete stimulus patterns at each ear can result in enhanced speech intelligibility by binaural listening. Bocca (1955) reported that in testing normal listeners with a low-level, high-fidelity signal to one ear while a high-level, low-pass reproduction was presented to the other ear, the dichotic (binaural) speech discrimination scores equalled the sum of their monaural discrimination scores for each version separately. Other investigators have obtained better discrimination for monosyllables when a high-pass filtered version was presented to one ear and a low-pass filtered version to the other ear, than when either ear received the signal monaurally. In fact, tests involving the ability of the auditory system to integrate or fuse filtered or distorted signals are often administered to determine if there is any central or temporal lobe abnormality. Distorted signals to each ear are normally integrated much more effectively than monaurally.

15 *Use of Split-Band Amplification in Binaural Hearing Aid Fittings*

Studies have been reported which have evaluated the effects of augmenting a high-frequency band with a low-frequency band and of the differences between presenting the low-frequency band to the same ear or to the opposite ear. Franklin (1975) reported the result of a study with persons having moderate-to-severe sensorineural hearing losses. A low-frequency passband of 240Hz-480Hz and a high-frequency passband of 1020Hz-2040Hz were presented to either the same or opposite ears of the hearing-impaired person. When the low-frequency band and the high-frequency band were added to the same ear, there was little change in the consonant recognition score, but, when presented to opposite ears, there was a significant increase in the score at each of three sensation levels used. It would appear that the increased discrimination for consonants resulted from the release of the masking effect of the low-frequency band on the high-frequency band when each band is presented to separate ears. When both bands are delivered to the same ear, there will be a peripheral masking effect of low-frequency components of speech on the high-frequency components of speech. Normally, the extent of this masking effect is dependent on the intensity level of the low-frequency signals. It is interesting to note that although Franklin observed differences dependent on the sensation levels when testing normal listeners, she reported significant differences between monaural and binaural discrimination scores for sensorineural listeners at all sensation levels. The results of her study have important implications for the bandwidth of the frequency response of hearing aids used for binaural fittings. It should be mentioned that recent investigations have indicated that the fusion effect is poorer in geriatrics than younger people. Therefore, specialists must be cautious about recommending split-band binaural hearing aid fittings for the presbyacusic population. Manufacturers of hearing aids should be encouraged to investigate different frequency responses for aids to be used in binaural fittings.

16 *Attitudinal Factors*

Several recent writers on binaural hearing aid fittings have suggested that the trend toward binaural amplification is as much a function of the dispensers' and the users' attitudes on the advantage of binaural as of the actual differences observed in performance between the monaural and binaural fitting (Mueller, 1986). It is true that the bias of the professional involved in the hearing aid selection process as well as the bias of the client will influence the final decision as to the mode of amplification. However, where it can be demonstrated through properly conducted sound-field audiometric testing that the binaural mode is more effective in providing better speech intelligibility or localization of sources of sound, it is possible often to overcome a negative attitude toward the use of two hearing aids. At least the specialist selecting the proper mode of amplification should enable a suitable candidate to judge if significant differences do exist in the use of the dichotic mode compared to the monaural.

As more research is conducted on binaural hearing aid fittings and the results published, it becomes more evident that the preponderance of bilaterally hearing-impaired individuals are good candidates for binaural fittings. However, everyone suffering from bilateral hearing dysfunction is not necessarily a good candidate for binaural amplification. The clinician responsible for making the final decision as to the proper mode of amplification has the responsibility of verifying binaural responses, preferably through soundfield audiometry. The subject should be carefully tested by the use of pure-tones, pulsed or warbled, and speech comparing the results from applicable modes of amplification.

CONTRAINDICATIONS TO BINAURAL HEARING AID FITTINGS

The following psychoacoustic factors can often be significant in recommending the use of monaural amplification rather than binaural:

1 *Degradation Effect*

When the results of speech discrimination score testing indicate excellent or a good score for one ear and a poor score for the other, the client must be tested binaurally to determine that amplification into the poorer ear does not result in degradation of the good hearing in the better ear. It is possible for amplification into a badly distorted ear to degrade the signal traveling through the auditory pathway from the better ear.

2 *Fusion or Integration Effect*

There are hearing-impaired persons suffering not only from peripheral hearing problems but also from central auditory dysfunction. In some cases, fusion of signals between the two ears may function so poorly that they receive better results when listening with only one ear. However, in many cases there has been a deprivation of binaural input for long periods of time and the individual may require a period of adaptation and adjustment to two eared hearing. In these cases, a trial period may be advantageous to see if such persons can eventually find binaural hearing aids more beneficial than monaural amplification.

3 *Dynamic Range*

Where one ear has a very small dynamic range, the binaural fitting may not be appropriate. In some cases it is very difficult to compress the dynamic range of speech into a very limited range of tolerance for changes in the amplitude of sound pressure. Then the ear with the wider dynamic range should normally be fitted.

4 *Diplacusis*

A person suffering from binaural diplacusis perceives the same pure-tone presented to each ear alternately as being of a different pitch. Because of this disorder of pitch perception, these individuals have proven poor candidates for binaural hearing aid fittings.

5 *Threshold of Discomfort*

A person with an unusually low threshold of discomfort in one ear can prove a poor subject for binaural amplification. Normally such individual would also have a very narrow dynamic range. This person probably would be more comfortable with an aid fitted to the ear with a higher threshold of discomfort and wider dynamic range for the reception of amplified speech.

6 *Psychological Factor in Binaural Hearing Aid Fittings*

There are those individuals among the hearing-impaired whose audiometric profile indicates a recommendation for binaural hearing aids. However, some individuals cannot tolerate the feeling resulting from both ears being occluded. They claim that they have a sensation of being 'closed in or confined'. They cannot be fitted binaurally.

7 *Physical Factors in Binaural Hearing Aid Fittings*

Hearing-impaired persons with multiple disabilities such as cases of cerebral palsy have motor dysfunction. It is difficult for them to handle one hearing aid properly. Then, there are also elderly people suffering from hearing loss who find handling one hearing aid a tremendous task; in such cases, two hearing aids would be overwhelming.

TESTS COMPARING BINAURAL AND MONAURAL HEARING AID FITTINGS

There are those in academia who have resisted the fitting of binaural hearing aids arguing that the tests have not as yet been developed to reveal the benefits of binaural over monaural listening. Those dispensers who have supported the two eared fitting have observed the results of improved speech discrimination and therefore better acceptance of hearing aids by their clients. In the interest of demonstrating such improvement in clinical testing, I have proposed the following procedures and geometric arrangements of loudspeakers in an acoustically treated sound field, as illustrated in Figure 5. At least three loudspeakers should be employed in the sound room, in order to avoid any head-shadow effect causing significant signal-to-noise ratio differences at the two ears as explained previously in this chapter. The person tested should be seated at a position in the room that is equidistant from each of the three loudspeakers. The signal-to-noise ratio should be + 5dB, with speech being presented through the center by the two lateral loudspeakers at sound pressure levels of 60dB, which should summate at the midline of the head at 63dB.

Use of the revised Peterson-Lehiste CNC words or the Duffy Phoneme Recognition Tests (listed in chapter VII by Duffy) is encouraged. A partial credit method of scoring should then be employed. Scoring of each correct phoneme is a finer measure of speech discrimination than the conventional all-or-nothing method of scoring each word correctly

Sound Field Structuring of Loudspeakers for Binaural Hearing Aid Testing

1. Geometric array of three or more speakers.
2. Independent noise sources for each lateral speaker.
3. Use Duffy Phonemic word Recognition List.
4. Failure of language development use Warble Tones.
5. Use partial credit scoring method.

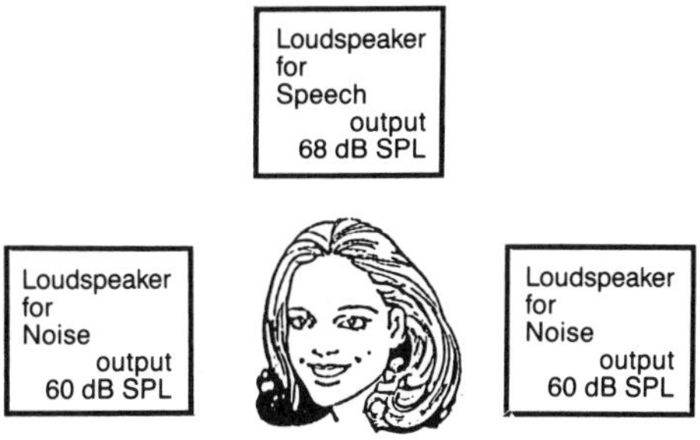

Loudspeaker for Speech output 68 dB SPL

Loudspeaker for Noise output 60 dB SPL

Loudspeaker for Noise output 60 dB SPL

| Speech | 68 dB |
| Noise | 63 dB |

| Signal to Noise Ratio | +5dB |

Fig. 5.

recognized. Very often differences between monaural and binaural modes of amplification will be elicited through phonemic scoring that would not be revealed using the conventional procedure.

B. *Monaural Mode of Amplification*

In fitting hearing aids for those hearing-impaired individuals for whom either the professional (physician, audiologist or hearing aid specialist) prefers monaural amplification or the client insists on wearing only one hearing aid, I suggest using the following guidelines in selecting the proper ear for amplification.

1 *Speech Discrimination*

Select the ear to be fitted with the hearing aid which indicates the better speech discrimination. The speech tests selected to evaluate the ability of each ear to discriminate speech should be sufficiently sensitive to elicit differences that may exist in each auditory pathway. Tests of speech discrimination are usually conducted under earphones in quiet. However, a competing acoustic stimulus or noise can often help indicate acuity differences between ears that are not apparent by testing in quiet. In addition, speech discrimination tests can be conducted in a soundfield by masking the non-test ear. In soundfield testing it is good practice to employ the client's customized earmold with the appropriate hearing aid to validate that the proper ear has been selected.

I further suggest that the phonemic (partial scoring for correct identification of phonemes) scoring method (Duffy, 1967) be employed as it is more sensitive than the conventional all-or-nothing method of scoring speech discrimination tests. It is further suggested that speech discrimination tests be conducted at presentation levels approximating the client's most comfortable loudness level (MCL). When discrimination tests are performed in a background of noise, I recommend using a signal-to-noise ratio of +5dB. It has been found that for sensorineural hearing losses of mild and moderate severity, a +5dB signal-to-noise ratio results in scores which do not cluster in such high percentages that the assessment of differences existing between ears becomes difficult.

I have used an 8% or greater difference in discrimination scores between the ears as a criterion in selecting the better ear for amplification. Normally, I have obtained good reliability on repeated speech tests comparing the function of each ear. Invariably, when I have made two earmolds and have asked the client to compare results of amplification in everyday life, they have preferred the ear which indicated better speech discrimination when tested in my office. However, the exception to the rule of fitting the better speech discriminating ear, would be those cases where the pure-tone average for speech reception thresholds in the better ear does not exceed 45dB HL and the speech discrimination score in the poorer ear is 80% or better, fitting the poorer ear should still result in good speech intelligibility and permit the contribution of auditory cues from the unaided better ear. In fact, those cases where discrimination scores are better than 80% in both ears and the pure-tone averages and speech reception thresholds in the better ear varies from 30dB to 45dB HL, I recommend making custom earmolds for both ears and advising the client to try wearing the aid in each ear. The client can be instructed to wear the hearing aid in the poorer ear when in a noisy environment, thus having a binaural advantage as the unaided better ear will still contribute auditory cueing. The client can be advised to wear the hearing aid in the better ear when in a quiet environment to obtain maximum speech discrimination. In fact, every effort should be made to convince the client to wear binaural aids.

2 Dynamic Range

The dynamic range (DR) of the ear has been defined as the difference between the threshold of discomfort (TD) and the speech reception threshold (SRT). When the determination of the ear to be fitted cannot be made based on speech discrimination scores, as such scores are approximately the same in each ear, then selection can be based on the ear with the larger dynamic range. I have maintained that a dynamic range of 50dB is required in an ear in order to accommodate the dynamic range of average speech. The difference between the strongest vowel (the aw sound) in English speech and the weakest consonant (the voiceless th sound) is approximately 28dB. Loud speech is approximately 10dB greater than average speech of 65dB SPL, and soft speech is approximately 10dB less than average speech, making a total difference of 20dB from soft to loud speech. Therefore, if we add the 28dB to the 20dB we have a total of 48dB as a required dynamic range to accommodate amplitude changes in speech. In accordance with this rationale, a dynamic range of approximately 50dB would be necessary for the auditory perception of changes in intensity of the acoustic wave form of soft and loud speech. The ear with the largest dynamic range should therefore be selected for the hearing aid fitting as it will better accommodate intensity changes which take place in everyday conversation.

If the dynamic range of the ear selected for use of a hearing aid is less than 40dB, compression amplification should be considered. When linear amplification is used with an impaired ear having a narrow dynamic range, the peaks of the speech wave form will often be clipped, resulting in a high percentage of harmonic distortion. The use of compression amplification in hearing aids can minimize harmonic distortion by presenting the dynamic range of speech within the dynamic range of the hearing-impaired ear fitted.

3   Threshold of Discomfort

Select the ear with the highest threshold of discomfort when selecting a monaural hearing aid and the speech discrimination scores are approximately the same in both ears. An ear with a higher threshold of discomfort can better tolerate the amplified signal from the hearing aid. It is important that the maximum pressure output of the hearing aid recommended not exceed the threshold of discomfort of the ear fitted in order to preserve both comfort and safety from further deterioration of the listener's hearing. In testing to determine the threshold of discomfort of an impaired ear, I have defined this level as one at which the loudness of the sound reaching the ear becomes annoying to the listener. Since an individual would normally reject wearing a hearing aid whose output is constantly exceeding an annoyance level, the maximum pressure output of an aid becomes the critical factor involved in selecting appropriate electroacoustic characteristics for amplification.

I have suggested that the measurement of the threshold of discomfort of an ear be conducted with speech as the acoustic stimulus. However, uncomfortable loudness levels at specific frequencies (250Hz, 500Hz, 1000Hz, 2000Hz and 4000Hz) or narrow bands of noise centering at such critical frequencies can be measured either under earphones or in a sound field.

4 *Conductive Component*

Normally the ear with the larger air-bone gap (conductive component) should be selected in a monaural fitting. The larger conductive component will usually result in a higher threshold of discomfort and a larger dynamic range for the ear. However, in fitting conductive or mixed hearing losses, one should be certain that there is no medical contra-indication to occluding a particular ear with a middle ear problem. Individuals suffering from conductive or mixed hearing losses having large conductive components will have good speech discrimination and usually accept amplification readily. In addition, the conductive component will prove a cushion for attenuation of louder sounds before reaching the cochlea of the ear. However, the conductive and mixed losses do require greater gain from the hearing aid which often necessitates tighter earmolds to avoid feedback or better sealing all-in-the-ear fittings.

5 *Flat Audiograms*

When the ear to be selected cannot be determined by the above mentioned criteria, a good rule to follow is select the ear with the flattest air conduction threshold audiogram for the monaural fitting. The ear with the flatter audiogram will enable many high-frequency components of speech to become audible and be heard at higher sensation levels than the descending or ski-slope audiometric configuration. This increase in audibility should be reflected in better speech discrimination with appropriate selective amplification. In the special case of an ear indicating a rising audiogram, the ear with the flatter audiogram should be fitted, since the ear with good high-frequency thresholds (the rising audiogram) will contribute many consonantal cues to overall speech intelligibility, even though it is unaided.

6 *70dB (ANSI) Rule*

This particular guideline for ear selection in a monaural fitting is probably one of the oldest criteria, and was formerly known, when the ASA, 1951 calibration standard was used for audiometers, as the 60dB Rule. As the change to the ANSI, 1969 calibration standard resulted in a change of approximately 10dB average increase of hearing levels, I have termed it the 70dB Rule. It actually consists of three separate recommendations:

a. When both ears indicate pure-tone air conduction averages (500Hz, 1000Hz and 2000Hz) or speech reception thresholds better than 70dB HL, fit the poorer ear.

b. When both ears indicate pure-tone air conduction averages (500Hz, 1000Hz and 2000Hz) or speech reception thresholds poorer than 70dB HL, fit the better ear.

c. When one ear indicates pure-tone air conduction average (500Hz, 1000Hz and 2000Hz) or speech reception threshold better than 70dB HL, and the other ear indicates pure-tone air conduction average (500Hz, 1000Hz and 2000Hz) or speech reception threshold poorer than 70dB HL, fit the ear with the pure-tone average or speech reception threshold closer to 70dB HL.

The 70dB Rule should only be applied when both ears indicate similar speech discrimination scores, dynamic ranges, thresholds of discomfort, air-bone gaps or sensorineural hearing losses and audiogram configurations.

7 *Tinnitus*

When the client suffers from unilateral tinnitus which often can be masked by the hearing aid and the ear has good speech discrimination, then this ear should be considered for the monaural hearing aid fitting. In fact, many clients with mild and moderate hearing losses are more concerned with their tinnitus than with their hearing loss and will accept the hearing aid if it provides a masking effect to their tinnitus. However, when an ear with tinnitus has very poor discrimination for speech, and the contralateral ear shows much better acuity for speech, then the professional responsible for the evaluation should insist on fitting the ear with the better intelligibility for speech and either a masker or hearing aid for the ear suffering from tinnitus.

8 *Client Preference*

In those cases where the audiometric data for both ears is very similar, I often prepare a mold for each ear and advise the client to try the aid selected in each ear and wear it predominantly in the ear which appears to give the best results in terms of speech intelligibility, comfortability and quality of sound. Where a client would prefer my selection of an ear to be fitted under the above circumstances, I am biased toward the right ear. Recent studies Kimura (1961) have reported a right ear and left hemisphere dominance for

speech. Since most people would have such right ear dominance and the audiometric tests are approximately the same
for both ears, I would like the person fitted to have the
advantage of this dominance effect in their use of the
hearing aid in everyday life.

9   *Quality of Hearing Aid User's Own Voice*

There are those hearing-impaired individuals who complain
that their own voices sound 'strange or reverberative' when
hearing through the hearing aid. This acoustic phenomenon
occurs as a result of the occlusion effect. The bone conduction threshold for low-frequency sounds is better by as
much as 20dB at 250Hz, 15dB at 500Hz and 10dB at
1000Hz by occluding the external canal. The only means of
persuading a client to accept the hearing aid is to loosen the
fit of the earmold and in many cases trying a non-occluding
earmold. However, normally when more than approximately 38dB of gain is required, a non-occluding type of
earmold may result in a feedback problem. If possible,
trying the other ear may result in satisfaction to the person
being fitted. An alternative, when more gain is required, is
the use of a CROS mode of amplification (the separation of
microphone on one side of the head from the receiver on the
other side of the head enables the use of non-occluding type
of earmold and with greater amount of gain without the
occurrence of feedback).

It has been my experience that venting of an occluded
earmold has not been that effective in eliminating the reverberative effect of the user's own voice. However, it is still
worth trying in those cases where more than 38dB of gain is
required and open or non-occluding earmolds will defi-
nitely result in feedback. When venting, a parallel vent is
preferred as it does not reduce the high-frequency response
of the aid as often happens with the branch vent.

10   *Physiological Factors in Ear Selection*

If an individual with a moderate to severe bilateral hearing
loss has a prolapsed canal in one ear and the other ear canal
is normal, the audiological data being similar in both ears,
fit the ear with the normal external canal, where an earmold
with proper sealing can be made (fitting the prolapsed canal
ear will often result in feedback when moderate or high
gain is required). In addition, the insertion of an occluding
mold into a prolapsed canal can often be annoying, if not
painful to many clients. If the loss is mild then a non-

occluding type of earmold can be employed. The non-occluding type of earmold will also avoid the loss of the natural resonance of the ear canal which can be as much as 21dB at 2700Hz.

There are ears in which the cartilage of the pinna is so soft or fragile that it will not support the weight of a postauricular hearing aid. If the audiometric results are approximately the same in both ears, select the ear with the firmer cartilage of the pinna. If not, an all-in-the-ear type of hearing aid should be considered. When fitting all-in-the-ear type of hearing aids, and audiometrically there is no significant difference between the two ears, select the ear in which the concha is larger and better recessed to accommodate the hearing aid physically.

The specialist must also consider the width of the ear canal in making a decision on the ear to be selected for the use of the hearing aid. There are ear canals that are extremely narrow such as in the case of small children and it is difficult to produce an earmold with sufficient occlusion where high-gain amplification is required.

C. Diotic (Y-cord) Mode of Amplification

The diotic mode of listening, as illustrated in Figure 3, refers to identical acoustic signals being delivered to each ear. There is no interaural difference in either phase, time, intensity, or frequency at the eardrums as the output of one hearing aid is split and presented to each ear. The diotic mode is often referred to as either the Y-cord mode or the pseudo-binaural mode of listening. The Y-cord which connects the amplifier to the two receivers can be designed so that the two transducers are either in parallel or in series. It is important for the specialist recommending a Y-cord arrangement to specify whether the system shall be in series or in parallel, as the output impedance of the receiver depends on the type of system employed.

The Y-cord arrangement has been recommended by clinicians as a temporary fitting when it has been impossible to establish reliable thresholds of hearing. Once reliable and valid hearing threshold levels have been established and there is a need for amplification, then a monaural or binaural fitting is preferred based on the audiometric evaluation.

It has been demonstrated by Black and Hast, (1962) that the diotic mode employed in an amplifying system in which the same acoustic signals were applied through earphones to the two ears had no increased effect on speech intelligibility. Their investigation revealed that mere duplication of acoustic information at each ear does not improve speech perception. There must be additional subtle cues resulting from differences in the acoustic waveforms at the ears for enhancement of speech intelligibility. Therefore, I have maintained that the Y-cord mode of amplification should be used only as a temporary fitting until such time as an accurate and reliable audiogram can be obtained. Once the clinician has determined that thresholds of hearing are valid, either binaural hearing aids or a monaural hearing aid can be recommended for proper amplification.

D. *CROS Mode of Amplification*

Historically, the first CROS hearing aid was designed to provide amplification for persons suffering from a unilateral hearing loss. Many of these cases had no aidable hearing in one ear, and normal or near-normal hearing in the other ear. They would complain of problems in localizing sources of sound and of poor speech discrimination when the source of speech was on the side of the poor ear. The head-shadow effect, previously explained in this chapter, would cause the high-frequency components of the speech signal to be attenuated significantly due to ineffective diffraction of such high-frequency sound waves in traveling around the head to the better ear. The average attenuation for speech in traveling from one ear, around the head to the other ear is normally 6dB-7dB. However, the high-frequency diminishment in intensity can be as great as 20dB. It occurred to some researchers such as Wallstein and Wigand (1962) and Harford and Barry (1965) that the placement of a microphone in or near the unaidable ear and routing the signal to the better ear would avoid the attenuation of high-frequency components of speech. Harford and Barry named the hearing aid with the microphone on the side of the unaidable ear and the amplifier and receiver on the side of the normal or aidable ear, contralateral routing of signal or CROS.

The use of CROS hearing aids, the signal being routed into an ear normal or close to normal, necessitated the selection of amplifiers with minimal gain requirements. In addition, the use of mild gain and mild output hearing aids permitted the employment of open or non-occluding types of earmolds, since there was seldom any feedback problem. There were many advantages derived from using tubings, open or non-occluding molds such as the preservation of normal ear canal resonance (this resonance peak at approximately 17dB-21dB at 2700Hz is lost when ear is occluded), improved comfortability and attenuation of low-frequencies (avoidance of masking effect of lows on high-frequencies).

TYPES OF UNAIDABLE EARS

1 An audiogram indicates profound sensorineural loss of such severity that it is improbable that audibility can be achieved in the ear with maximum amplification.

2 An ear with severe or profound mixed loss suffering from atresia (absence of any normal anatomical opening) of the ear canal; the sensorineural component of hearing loss being so large that bone conduction is not feasible.

3 An ear with an abnormally small dynamic range (threshold of discomfort 105dB and speech reception threshold 100dB, dynamic range 5dB). It would be impossible to compress the dynamic range of speech into such a small dynamic range of the pathological ear.

4 An ear that indicates an abnormally low threshold of discomfort and therefore would be unable to tolerate amplified speech.

5 An ear with very poor speech discrimination would not be helped appreciably with amplification and may even degrade the better speech discrimination of the better ear.

6 An ear which is being treated medically or the otolaryngologist recommends that amplification for such ear be avoided.

CLASSIC CROS

PURE TONE AUDIOGRAM

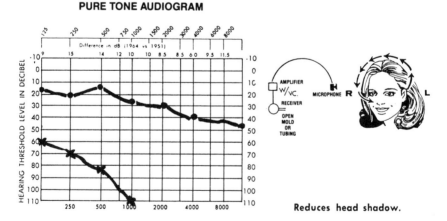

Reduces head shadow.

Fig. 6.

Although, the original intent of CROS hearing aids was for the unilateral hearing loss, over the years many other applications have been suggested and are being utilized:

1 *Classic CROS*

The classic CROS with microphone positioned on the side of the unaidable ear and amplifier and receiver on side of the better ear, using an open mold has had its best results and acceptance with cases that show a very mild high-frequency loss in the good ear (see Figure 6).

2 *Mini-CROS*

The mini CROS with microphone positioned on the side of the unaidable ear and amplifier and receiver on the side of the better ear, no mold being used at all, the receiver nozzle from the hearing aid is simply directed towards the better ear. It is used where the threshold of hearing for one ear is completely normal at all frequencies tested (see Figure 7).

3 *Uni-CROS*

One side of aid contains microphone, amplifier and receiver, occluding earmold directs amplified sound into aidable ear. This hearing aid is connected to amplifier and receiver on contralateral side of head, an open earmold delivers sound to better ear. Since acoustic signal is being amplified into both ears through only one

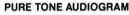

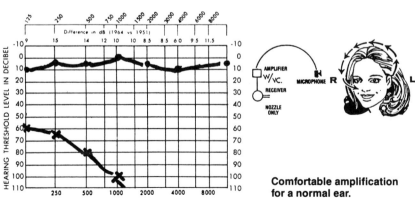

Comfortable amplification for a normal ear.

Fig. 7.

microphone the advantage of such system is questionable. I would recommend binaural hearing aid fittings in such cases where the client could have the advantage of additional auditory cues rather than splitting the output as suggested with uni-CROS (see Figure 8).

4 *Multi-CROS*

The multi-CROS is a very flexible hearing aid (see Figure 9). Through the use of a three way switch it is possible to produce either a monaural hearing aid, a CROS hearing aid or a BICROS hearing aid. Either open or occluding earmold can be used with a multi-CROS system dependent on the severity of the hearing loss in the ear to which the sound is directed.

5 *IROS*

IROS, ipsilateral routing of signal, means that a tubing, open or non-occluding earmold is employed. The correct terminology should be monaural or a binaural fitting. One has to be careful with open mold fittings in the amount of gain being delivered through the aid to an ear where moderate to high gain is required, as acoustic feedback may result. The microphone and receiver are both located on the same side of the head (see Figure 10) and the proximity of the two transducers can often cause a feedback problem where the gain exceeds 38dB in an open mold fitting.

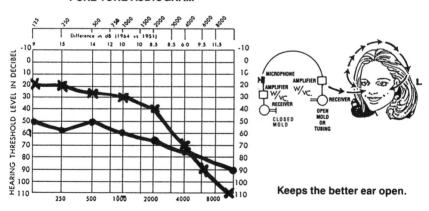

Keeps the better ear open.

Fig. 8.

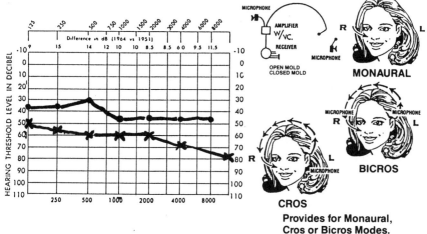

PURE TONE AUDIOGRAM

MONAURAL

BICROS

CROS

Provides for Monaural,
Cros or Bicros Modes.

Fig. 9.

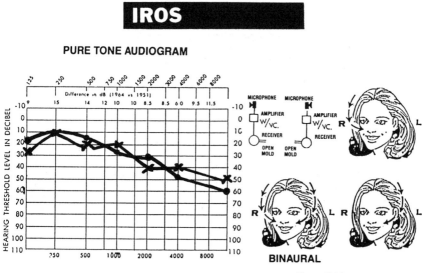

PURE TONE AUDIOGRAM

BINAURAL

For mild loss.

Fig. 10.

6 *Focal CROS*

The focal CROS is very similar to the classic CROS having the microphone positioned on the unaidable side and the amplifier and receiver positioned at the side of the better ear using an open earmold. However, the focal CROS has a tube extending from the microphone to the pinna of the unaidable ear. It has been suggested that receiving the acoustic signal in close vicinity of the ear canal enhances the high-frequency response (see Figure 11).

7 *Power CROS*

Power CROS is used for severe hearing loss, enabling those hearing-impaired who require high-gain and high-power output hearing aids to avoid acoustic feedback problem. By having the microphone positioned on one side of the head and the receiver on the other side, we can obtain additional output without feedback due to the separation. Therefore, an occluding earmold is used with the power CROS (see Figure 12).

8 *High CROS*

High CROS is used for a bilateral high-frequency hearing loss. The use of an open mold fitting enables the reduction of the low-frequency components of speech where hearing thresholds are good. The separation of microphone and receiver enables the hearing-impaired individual to obtain higher gain in the high-frequencies without acoustic feedback (see Figure 13).

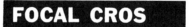

PURE TONE AUDIOGRAM

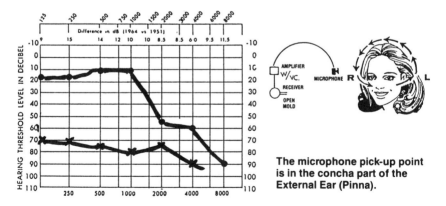

The microphone pick-up point is in the concha part of the External Ear (Pinna).

Fig. 11.

POWER CROS

PURE TONE AUDIOGRAM

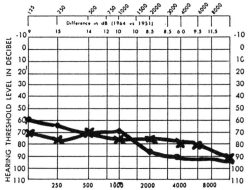

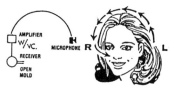

Separation of microphone
and receiver avoids feedback.

Fig. 12.

HIGH CROS

PURE TONE AUDIOGRAM

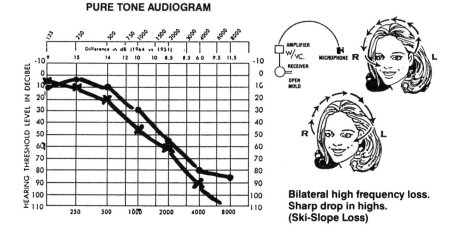

Bilateral high frequency loss.
Sharp drop in highs.
(Ski-Slope Loss)

Fig. 13.

9 *BICROS*

BICROS contains two microphones, one positioned on each side
of the head. The output of each microphone is directed to one
amplifier and one receiver using either an non-occluding or

occluding earmold dependent on the severity of the hearing loss in the better ear (see Figures 14 and 15). BICROS has not been extensively used as many users have complained of interference with the signal from the aid on the better ear. I believe this is due to the fact that an individual wearing a BICROS tends to position the better ear toward the source of sound and thereby receives

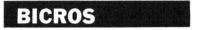

PURE TONE AUDIOGRAM

Two sided hearing from one hearing aid.

Fig. 14.

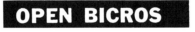

PURE TONE AUDIOGRAM

When mild gain is indicated.

Fig. 15.

additional ambient noise through the microphone on the contralateral side.

CROS and BICROS hearing aids have declined in use since the advent of the all-in-the-ear and all-in-the-canal type of hearing aids. When eyeglass temple hearing aids were popular CROS and BICROS aids were being recommended since it was quite convenient to conceal the wiring connecting the microphone to the amplifier in the zyl frame of the eyeglass. With all-in-the-ear type of hearing aids the use of CROS and BICROS requires the wiring connecting the microphone and amplifier to be placed behind the head, often under the hair. Many clients object to wearing a hearing aid in this manner as they claim the wiring behind the head annoys them. There are manufacturers of hearing aids producing CROS and BICROS modes of amplification without the use of wiring. These aids make use of radio frequency transmission and the manufacturers of such aids receive permission from the Federal Communications Commission to transmit on assigned ultra high-frequency bands. The wireless CROS and BICROS is available in post-auricular shells.

BONE CONDUCTION HEARING AID FITTINGS

Most experienced specialists involved in the selection of hearing aids would prefer to fit air conduction rather than the bone conduction type of amplifiers. I only recommend bone conduction type of fitting for mild or moderate conductive hearing losses suffering from either bilateral atresia (no ear canals) or chronic discharging ears. Even with those individuals who have a history of chronic discharge due to persistent draining otitis media, I recommend making (non-occluding where possible) earmolds for both ears and encourage the client to use the hearing aid alternately until the condition subsides.

In my opinion, audiometric threshold tests should indicate an average air-bone gap of approximately 40dB for the critical frequencies of 500Hz, 1000Hz and 2000Hz before a bone conduction type of amplifier is recommended.

An acoustic signal transmitted by bone conduction through the bones of the head will stimulate both cochleae.

However, there will be differences in the conductivity of the acoustic signal dependent upon the amount of fatty tissue covering an individual's mastoid process. Also, the curvature of the surface of the bone at the temporal process behind the ear will affect the conductivity of the acoustic stimulus. Therefore, the bone oscillator should be applied to each mastoid process and the side which produces the best auditory response should be the one used. Normally, this will be the particular mastoid of the ear which indicates the larger air-bone gap in audiometric testing.

Since it requires an additional 40dB of sound pressure through a bone oscillator for equal loudness for a similar acoustic signal heard by air conduction, much greater gain and output is needed for bone conduction fittings. I have found the most appropriate bone conduction fittings to be the use of a body hearing aid with the oscillator being applied against the mastoid bone by a metal headband. The eyeglass or headband type of hearing aid used with a bone conduction oscillator normally provides minimum pressure resulting in poor hearing response due to poor transmission. In those cases where the client refuses to use a body aid, several manufacturers have designed special high-gain postauricular hearing aids with bone oscillators using steel headbands. It has been my experience that this type of bone conduction fitting results in better response than the eyeglass bone conduction amplifier. There are also more problems of acoustic feedback with eyeglass bone conduction hearing aids when the gain is sufficient to present speech at preferred listening levels. I would therefore limit the recommendation of eyeglass bone conduction hearing aids to the mild conductive loss of hearing.

SUMMARY

The hearing aid specialist's decision as to the mode of amplification is critical in hearing aid selection. The availability of monaural, binaural, Y-cord, CROS and BICROS enables the professional to select the appropriate mode based on the client's audiometric profile, vocational and social needs.

This chapter has listed and explained the psychoacoustic advantages of the available modes of amplification. The benefits of binaural hearing aid fittings have been stressed as a means of achieving maximum speech discrimination for most hearing-impaired. In addition, binaural hearing aids should help the person suffering from a bilateral hearing loss to structure auditory space properly. This often results in a satisfied hearing aid user and a successful fitting.

Where the audiometric information indicates a monaural fitting is applicable, this chapter has listed and described rules for the selection of the ear to be fitted. The guidelines for monaural fittings has resulted in better use and acceptance of the hearing aid.

Hearing losses where one ear is unaidable can often be helped by the CROS mode of amplification with its many variations or by the use of BICROS.

The limited use for the bone conduction type of hearing aid has been explained.

It would appear that with the variety of modes of amplification and different electroacoustic performance characteristics available in hearing aids, appropriate amplification for all types of losses can be selected and the acoustic needs of the hearing-impaired satisfied.

GLOSSARY

Antiphasic conditions This condition exists when the speech signal at the two ears is in phase and the noise signal at the two ears is out of phase, or when the speech signal at the two ears is out of phase and the noise signal at the two ears is in phase.

BICROS mode of amplification One complete hearing aid and one custom earmold is fitted to a moderately impaired ear, connected to an additional microphone placed on the side of the severely deafened ear.

Bilateral mode of amplification One hearing aid containing one microphone and one amplifier but two cords and two receivers. The output from the amplifier is split to the two ears (Y-cord arrangement). It may be designed with a separate volume control for each receiver.

Binaural mode of amplification Two complete and independent hearing aids, one for each ear. This arrangement employs two separate transmission systems each containing one microphone, amplifier and receiver.

Binaural masking level differences (BMLD) The difference in the level of the acoustic signal for detection between two binaural conditions. A reversal of phase, in either the speech signal or the noise signal resulting in an antiphasic condition can change the binaural threshold in the low-frequencies significantly.

CROS mode of amplification The contralateral routing of signals, is a hearing aid system whereby the microphone of the hearing aid is placed on the side of the severely impaired ear and the amplifier and receiver are placed on the side of the normal or mildly impaired ear. The acoustic signal is normally routed into the better ear through an open or non-occluding mold.

Dichotic mode of amplification An arrangement, normally binaural hearing aids, whereby both ears are stimulated with acoustic signals simultaneously resulting in interaural differences in phase, time, intensity or frequency.

Diotic (pseudo-binaural, bilateral or Y-cord) mode of amplification The acoustic stimulus is applied to the two ears through one amplifying system resulting in similar information at each ear. There is no difference in intensity, time, phase or frequency, the acoustic stimulus is merely duplicated.

Head shadow effect The effect resulting from the interposition of the head to a source of sound which causes the high-frequency components of a complex signal to be attenuated. The low-frequency components of the signal are diffracted around the head much better than the high-frequency sounds. There can be as great as a 13dB change of signal-to-noise ratios existing at the two ears as a result of the head shadow effect.

Lateralization The sensation of hearing a sound in one ear rather than the other or the perception of movement of phantom auditory image across the head due to interaural differences in time, phase or intensity.

Localization The ability to judge the location of sound sources in terms of azimuth, elevation and distance resulting from interaural differences in phase, time, or intensity at the two ears. Localization refers to locating sources of sound external to the head whereas lateralization refers to an auditory image within the head itself.

Monotic mode of amplification This arrangement exists when an acoustic signal is amplified only to one ear, utilizing either one channel or two channel amplifying systems to that ear. When only one channel is utilized for amplification, it is a monaural amplifying system.

Squelch effect The ability of the auditory system to selectively listen to a desired acoustic stimulus and at the same time minimizing the effects of ambient noise. This selective listening is enhanced by the use of both ears through binaural hearing aids.

Summation effect The increase in the sensation of loudness through listening with two ears compared to hearing with one ear. At threshold, the summation effect for loudness is about 3dB, however at supra-thresholds of 30 to 35dB above threshold the summation effect can be approximately 6dB.

REFERENCES

BARFORD, J. (1979): "Speech perception processes and fitting of hearing aids." *Audiology*, 18, pp. 430-441.

BEGGS, W. D. A. & FOREMAN, D. L. (1980): "Sound localization and early binaural experience in the deaf." *British Journal of Audiology*, 14, pp. 41-48.

BERGMAN, M. (1957): "Binaural hearing." *Archives of Otolaryngol.*, 66, pp. 572-578.

BLACK, J. W. & HAST, M. H. (1962): "Speech reception with a hearing signal." *Journal of Speech and Hearing Research*, 5, pp. 70-75.

BOCCA, E. (1955): "Binaural hearing: another approach." *Laryngoscope*, 65, pp. 1164-1171.

BRISKEY, R. J. (1972): "Binaural hearing and new innovations." In J. Katz (Ed.) *Handbook of Clinical Audiology*. Williams and Wilkens Co., Baltimore, Md.

BROADBENT, D. E. (1956): "Growing points in multichannel communication." *Journal of Acoustical Society of America*, 28, pp. 533-535.

CAUSSE, R. & CHAVASSE, P. (1942): "Differences between binaural hearing threshold and monaural threshold for perception of super threshold intensities" (French) *Societe de Biologie et de les Filiales*, p. 136.

DUFFY, J. K. (1967): "Audio-visual speech audiometry and a new audio and audio-visual speech perception index." *Maico Acoustical Library Series*, 5, Report 9.

FRANKLIN, B. (1975): "The effect of combining low- and high-frequency passbands on consonant recognition in the hearing-impaired." *Journal of Speech and Hearing Research*, 18, pp. 719-727.

HARFORD, E. & BARRY, J. (1965): "A rehabilitation approach to the problem of unilateral hearing impairment, the contralateral routing of signals (CROS)." *Journal of Speech and Hearing Disorders*, 30, pp. 121-138.

HARRIS, J. D. (1965): "Monaural and binaural speech intelligibility and the stereophonic effect based upon temporal cues." *Laryngoscope*, 75, pp. 428-446.

JOHNSON, J. H. (1975): "Binaural hearing instrument system—the BiPhasic." *Hearing Instruments*, July pp. 20-21.

KILLION, M. C. (1982): "Transducers, earmolds and sound quality considerations." In G. A. Studebaker and F. H. Bess, (Eds.), The Vanderbilt Hearing-Aid Report, *Monographs in Contemporary Audiology*, Upper Darby, Pa., pp. 104-111.

KIMURA, D. (1961): "Cerebral dominance and perception of verbal stimuli." *Canad J. Psych.*, 15, pp. 166-171.

KOENIG, W. (1950): "Subjective effects in binaural hearing." *Journal of Acoustical Society of America*, 22, pp. 61-62.

LICKLIDER, J. C. (1948): "The influence of interaural phase relations upon the masking of speech by white noise." *Journal of Acoustical Society of America*, 20, pp. 150-159.

MARKIDES, A. (1977): "Binaural Hearing Aids." New York Academic Press.

MUELLER, H. G. (1986): "Binaural amplification: attitudinal factors." *The Hearing Journal*, 39, November, pp. 7-10.

NABELEK, A. K. (1982): "Temporal distortions and noise considerations." In G. A. Studebaker and F. H. Bess (Eds.), The Vanderbilt Hearing-Aid Report, *Monographs in Contemporary Audiology*, Upper Darby, Pa., pp. 51-59.

NABELEK, A. K. & PICKETT, J. M. (1974): "Reception of consonants in a classroom as affected by monaural and binaural listening, noise, reverberation and hearing aids." *Journal of Acoustical Society of America*, 56, pp. 628-639.

PETERSON, G. E. & LEHISTE, I. (1962): "Revised CNC lists for auditory tests." *Journal of Speech and Hearing Disorders*, 27, pp. 62-70.

SILMAN, S., GELFANT, S. A. & SILVERMAN, C. A. (1984): "Late-onset auditory deprivation: effects of monaural versus binaural hearing aids." *Journal of Acoustical Society of America*, 76, pp. 1357-1362.

TILLMAN, T. W., KASTEN, R. N. & HORNER, J. S. (1963): "Effect of head shadow on reception of speech." Paper read before American Speech and Hearing Association Convention. *Abstract ASHA*, 5, p. 778.

WULLSTEIN, H. L. & WIGAND, M. E. (1962): "A hearing aid for single ear deafness and its requirements." *Acta Otolaryngol.*, 54, pp. 136-142.

WESTERMANN, S. & TOPHOLM, J. (1985): "Comparing BTEs and ITEs for localizing speech." *Hearing Instruments*, February, pp. 20-24, 36.

ZELNICK, E. (1970): "Comparison of speech perception utilizing monotic and dichotic modes of listening." *Journal of Auditory Research*, 10, pp. 87-97.

ZELNICK, E. (1980): "The importance of interaural auditory differences in binaural hearing." In E. R. Libby (Ed.), *Binaural Amplification*, Zenetron, Inc., Chicago, Ill., pp. 81-103.

III

A PRESCRIPTIVE METHOD FOR HEARING AID SELECTION

KENNETH W. BERGER

INTRODUCTION

In 1972 we began working on a prescriptive hearing aid fitting procedure at Kent State University. These efforts resulted in a preliminary
published report a few years later Berger (1976), and summaries of the
procedure have appeared in print Berger (1978-1979-1980-1981). The
procedure encompasses (a) hearing aid candidacy, (b) whether the
right, left, or both ears should be fitted, (c) whether air or bone
conduction should be employed, (d) the prescription proper, and (e)
aided follow-up testing to determine how closely the fitted hearing aid's
response comes to that which was prescribed.

Observations of and comments from persons who fit hearing aids
suggest that older fitting methods are rapidly being replaced by prescriptive methods. It is, therefore, important to find out what prescriptive procedures consist of, as well as some of their strengths and
weaknesses in comparison with older fitting protocols.

CHAPTER OBJECTIVES

A series of orderly steps is appropriate in any hearing aid fitting
method. In the case of hearing aid prescription these steps are, presum-
ably, more specific and the results more readily testable than in other

fitting methods. In this chapter a particular hearing aid prescriptive method, often referred to as The Berger Method, will be considered. The focus will be on the rationale for the steps in this particular method, the actual procedures involved, and finally a brief summary of some results which we and others have obtained with the method.

PRELIMINARY STEPS TO THE PRESCRIPTION

In any hearing aid fitting method — excepting outright guessing! — it is to be expected that the specialist will follow an orderly series of decisions in arriving at the particular hearing aid which is selected, and with making the fitting itself. First, it is assumed that if there is a possibility that the hearing loss could be corrected by medicine or surgery the client will have that opportunity. Next, from audiometric test data the specialist will determine whether the logical fitting is to be for the right, left, or both ears, and whether an air- or bone-conduction fitting should be made. We have published guidelines on some of these topics (Berger & Millin, 1980) (Berger & Hagberg, 1982) (Berger & Hagberg, 1984), but they are not part of the actual prescription. Nonetheless, there are considerable differences of opinions among experienced clinicians on these subjects.

WHAT TO AMPLIFY

Assuming that the specialist has followed a standard set of decisions for the foregoing, the next question involves WHAT is to be amplified. It should not need stating that the hearing aid does not change the hearing mechanism, although it is surprising how often misinformation is found on the subject. That is, the hearing aid does not alter the tympanic membrane, the ossicles, the cochlea, or any part of the hearing system. Rather, the hearing aid accepts an external acoustic signal — specifically, and most importantly, speech — modifies that external signal, and delivers the modified signal to an ear that is just as impaired as it was previously. Although the hearing aid wearer may wish to hear birds sing again, or be able to better enjoy some form of music, the overriding reason for most people in obtaining a hearing aid is to improve their reception of and understanding of speech. It follows almost as an axiom, therefore, that the amplified signal should be closely related to, but a modification of, the incoming speech signal.

A number of scientifically determined models have been published which picture and describe the energy residing in typical speech. Most of these models use 65 dB SPL (45 dB HL) as the level of "average" speech at a distance of one meter between talker and listener. In addition, you and I, as well as those with hearing impairment, need to be able to hear and understand softer than average speech as well as louder than average speech. Although the energy in soft speech is about 55 dB SPL, average speech 65 dB SPL, and loud speech 75 dB SPL, actually the energy varies plus and minus 12 dB within each of those levels. More importantly, the various audio frequencies do not equally contribute to the intelligibility of speech. For example, we know from some early work by Harvey Fletcher at Bell Telephone Laboratories that the vowels and voiced consonants produce a lot of low-frequency energy but vowels contribute relatively little to discrimination of speech. In contrast, the consonants, especially the voiceless variety, are represented in the high-frequencies and contribute relatively little to the overall energy in the speech signal, however, they are highly important to word discrimination (Berger, 1980) (Berger, Klich, Millin, 1982).

But a moments reflection will confirm that this speech signal is arriving at all listeners. It is the same incoming signal for normal hearing individuals and for hearing impaired persons, for children and for the aged, for men and for women. Nor is there evidence that the relative energy in speech varies substantially whether the speaker is male or female, English speaking or using another modern language.

From the preceding it may be seen that, for ALL hearing aid wearers, it is logical to shape the amplified signal in reference to the speech spectrum. The speech spectrum shows a slight, gradual, increase of energy present in speech from the fundamental frequency of a person's voice (roughly 250 Hz for males and 325 Hz for females, but depending upon the specific vowels under consideration) up to a small peak at 500 or 550 Hz. Above that frequency the energy in speech gradually decreases to zero decibels at about 10,000 Hz (6, 22). From this, one can infer that the amplification of the higher frequencies, especially around 2000 to 3000 or 4000 Hz, is of utmost importance for the understanding of speech, while amplification of the lower frequencies is of considerably lesser importance for speech understanding, although the absence of amplification at the lower frequencies may sound quite artificial. Furthermore, it may easily be argued that much amplification of the lower frequencies is undesirable because the sounds from many background noises (motors, traffic, etc.) are in that frequency range and are distracting to understanding if not actually a cause of masking of the more important frequency ranges.

As has been seen, the energy in speech decreases rather significantly from octave to octave above 500 Hz. Unfortunately hearing loss patterns are most commonly such that the sensitivity decreases in that same range. Thus, one can readily appreciate how the person with more than a marginal hearing loss has difficulty with understanding consonants and, hence, word discrimination in general is reduced. All of this, of course, creates an impairment in receptive communication.

Accepting the foregoing, it follows that one cannot continue to increase the amount of amplification in the higher frequencies indefinitely. That is, since the energy present in speech decreases just as the hearing loss increases, it is inappropriate to completely mirror the speech spectrum by amplification. The old concept of "pure" selective amplification proposed doing something similar to that, but was unsuccessful because the gain in the low frequencies was usually more than appropriate, and in the higher frequencies was for the most part impossible to obtain. Furthermore, if it were possible to obtain enough gain in the higher frequencies to make up for the hearing loss, the large amount of amplification needed surely would have introduced further distortion into a hearing mechanism which already was, by definition, distorted. Thus, while it appears appropriate to use the speech spectrum as a model for shaping the amplified signal, the greater the hearing loss the less can the energy present in the higher frequencies of speech be adequately amplified above the hearing threshold level.

THE PRESCRIPTION BASELINE

Assuming now that an incomplete mirroring of the speech spectrum will be used as a pattern for the amplified signal, the next decision is where to anchor the prescription. That is, some audiometric base is needed on which to hinge the prescription. There are three fairly logical points for anchorage: the client's hearing threshold (HTL), most comfortable loudness level (MCL), and uncomfortable loudness level (UCL), or some arbitrary place between two of these.

There seems little question that the majority of hearing aid prescriptions — in fact hearing aid fittings by any formal method — directly involve the MCL. Despite being in the minority on this point, I strongly favor the client's threshold of sensitivity for the baseline of the prescription.

This is not to suggest that the hearing aid will be used at threshold, but merely that the threshold is the most stable of all routine audiometric test results and for prescriptive purposes has advantages. Just as importantly, if any behavioral audiometric test results can be obtained from an individual, it will be the threshold. To evaluate an individual's hearing the specialist may need to use a pediatric test such as COR or TROCA, or possibly even BSER, in which case thresholds are much more likely to be obtained than any other test results. For many small children, those with physical or mental problems, and even adults with normal intelligence, the task of signalling a reliable MCL is difficult

(Christen, Byrne, 1980) (Berger, Saltisz, 1981) (Berger, Abel, Hagberg, La Puzz, Varavvas & Weldele, 1982) (Berger, Hagberg, Varavvas & Vottero, 1982) (Berger, Varavvas & Vottero, 1982). Some dispensers argue that it is not difficult to obtain an MCL with most clients. With this I agree. What is difficult is to obtain a repeatable MCL. If one is to use a prescriptive hearing aid fitting method, reasonably precise and repeatable audiometric test measures are required. It is illogical to use precise prescriptive data based upon imprecise audiometric test results. There is considerable experimental evidence that the most comfortable *level* is actually a most comfortable *range*. Although the most comfortable range presents a nice wide target area for fitting, unfortunately it is not sufficiently precise for prescriptive purposes. Despite this, our particular goal will be to place the amplified signal within the person's comfortable loudness range, that is, above threshold insofar as is feasible, but below UCL. For this purpose HTL data will be employed for the prescription.

Like MCLs, word discrimination scores do not have adequate test-retest reliability for prescriptive purposes. The classical study by Shore, Bilger and Hirsh was the first of a number of published experimental studies to document word discrimination test variability (Shore, Bilger & Hirsh, 1960). Meanwhile efforts to improve word discrimination testing have appeared, such as presenting the words in noise, changing the method of scoring words missed, and changing words within lists so as to make them more homogenous. These efforts have often resulted in some increase in sensitivity of the tests but to our knowledge no evidence has been published to the effect that these alterations permit better test-retest reliability. Although our method does not employ speech audiometry for prescriptive purposes it will be noticed that most factors involved in the procedures are based upon speech acoustics.

AMOUNT OF AMPLIFICATION

To briefly summarize up to this point, we have decided to shape the amplified signal so as to mirror, insofar as is considered practical, the speech spectrum. The shaped signal will be anchored to the client's hearing threshold level, and later the nearness of the fitting result to the prescription can be determined by obtaining an aided threshold. We now need to consider the amount of amplification to be prescribed.

At this point let us determine how much gain is to be prescribed. In the 1950's Samuel F. Lybarger published what has become known as "the one-half gain rule". The one-half gain rule simply states that persons with a sensorineural hearing loss will tend to set the control of their hearing aid so as to supply gain amounting to one-half of the hearing loss. Thus, persons who have a 60 dB hearing threshold level will, for most listening environments, choose gain of 30 dB. Since the publication by Lybarger a number of studies in the United States and abroad have confirmed the validity of the one-half gain rule (Millin, 1965) (McCandless, Miller, 1972) (Martin, 1973) (Brooks, 1973) (Byrne, Fifield, 1974) (Morris, 1977) (Berger, Hagberg & Rane, 1980). I am unaware of any published data to refute the one-half gain rule.

There are, of course, a number of reasons why hearing aid wearers may set their hearing aid to produce gain of less than one-half of their hearing threshold level, but the ideal remains that of one-half gain. For example, if loud amplified sounds are uncomfortable to the hearing aid wearer because of an SSPL that is too high it is likely that the gain will be turned down in an effort to avoid those uncomfortably loud sounds. Or, if when the gain of the instrument is turned up to provide one-half of the hearing threshold level an acoustic feedback problem appears, obviously the gain will be reduced to below the feedback level.

In some ways, the overall amount of gain to be prescribed is of lesser importance than the saturation sound pressure level (SSPL), which will briefly be discussed below, or the shape of the amplified signal. The shape of the amplified signal is presumed to be directly related to speech intelligibility, whereas the amount of gain chosen can be readily increased or decreased by the wearer, depending upon the magnitude of the desired input signal, the amount of undesired background noise, or merely personal preference. It follows that the wearer should have some freedom in increasing or decreasing the gain — although hopefully not do so too often — depending upon the particular communication situation.

At this point the heart of our prescription can be put into a formula, as follows:

$$\frac{\text{HTL at 500 Hz}}{2} \; ; \; \frac{\text{HTL at 1000 Hz}}{1.6} \; ; \; \frac{\text{HTL at 2000 Hz}}{1.5}$$

$$\frac{\text{HTL at 3000 Hz}}{1.7} \; ; \; \frac{\text{HTL at 4000 Hz}}{1.9} \; ; \; \frac{\text{HTL at 6000 Hz}}{2}$$

This formula represents OPERATING GAIN. Operating gain is not the gain portion of the prescription, but rather the basis for plotting (that is, predicting) what the aided response should be. If all of the denominators in the formula were a "2" this would correspond to the one-half gain rule. Since some of the denominators are smaller than 2 the overall gain will be a little more than 50%. The peak of the gain, as can be seen, will be at 2000 Hz, which has been found in a number of studies to be the most important single frequency for speech understanding.

Having determined the operating gain, the desired aided response can next be plotted. For example, if the unaided hearing threshold level in the ear to be fitted was 60 dB at all test frequencies the operating gain would be 30 dB at 500 Hz, 38 dB at 1000 Hz, 40 dB at 2000 Hz, 35 dB at 3000 Hz, 32 dB at 4000 Hz, and if 6000 Hz is a frequency to be prescribed it would be 30 dB. Gain, of course, means that the aided threshold should be better by the magnitude of that operating gain. In this example the aided hearing threshold level target would be 30 dB at 500 Hz, 22 dB at 1000 Hz, 20 dB at 2000 Hz, 25 dB at 3000 Hz, 28 dB at 4000 Hz, and 30 dB at 6000 Hz. The audiogram could at this point be so marked, so that when the client is later tested while wearing the chosen hearing aid it can easily be visualized whether the predicted and obtained gain are closely related.

THE GAIN PRESCRIPTION

Operating gain, as noted, is not the prescription. Operating gain is not a standard term, it is only what you and I agree it should be. MAXIMUM GAIN is the first half of the prescription. Maximum gain is a standard term, understood by manufacturers and clinicians alike. Maximum Gain = Operating Gain + Reserve Gain ± correction factors to account for the microphone location (in-the-ear, behind-the-ear, on the body), and whether there is a conductive component to the hearing loss (in which case 1/5 of the air-bone gap will be added to the operating gain and to the maximum gain), and if this is a binaural fitting (in which case 3 dB will be subtracted from the maximum gain in appropriately chosen cases for that fitting). The correction factors for conductive losses and for binaural fittings are based upon experimental results (Berger, 1980) (Berger, Millin, 1980) (Domoracki, Berger & Millin, 1982) (Berger, 1984).

The correction factors, depending upon the microphone location, in turn, will be different if we are using technical data which were determined from hearing aid measurements made in the 2cc coupler or in the Zwislocki coupler on the manikin KEMAR®. Present ANSI standards involve the 2cc coupler, so that is what we have been using pending an updating of standards to another coupler.

For in-the-ear hearing aids the operating gain formula plus an arbitrary amount of reserve gain (we use 10 dB) will approximate the desired gain. Some specialists prefer to add a little extra gain at 2000, 3000, and 4000 Hz. For behind-the-ear hearing aids the loss of the pinna effect suggests adding 2 dB of gain at 2000 Hz and 3 dB at 3000

Hz, although, again, the specialist may want to add a little more at those higher frequencies. For body aids we reduce the maximum gain at 500 Hz and increase it at 2000 Hz in reference to that for in-the-ear aids, in an effort to partially overcome the body baffle effect. Whatever amount of maximum gain is prescribed, and whether from data obtained with the 2cc coupler or other coupler, one is dealing with technical data from measurements presented in printed specifications which are average, and it is often necessary for some adjustments to be made to the amplifier when fitted to a person.

SATURATION SOUND PRESSURE LEVEL

The second half of the prescription is that of SATURATION SOUND PRESSURE LEVEL (SSPL). In the older specification sheets and standards this was referred to as Output. For hearing aid selection purposes SSPL can be logically divided into two parts: Maximum Permissible SSPL and Minimum Desirable SSPL. The former is, of course, the most critical of the two since Maximum Permissible SSPL is designed to preclude amplified sounds from exceeding the client's uncomfortable loudness level (UCL). Obviously, a person will not continue to wear a hearing aid if sound is routinely amplified so as to be uncomfortably loud (Berger, 1976) (Berger, Rane & Hagberg, 1979).

To prescribe the Maximum Permissible SSPL the client's UCLs are obtained with discrete frequency signals. We use pulsing tones at 500, 1000, 2000, and 4000 Hz for this purpose. A standard set of instructions as well as procedures should be used for this determination because the UCL is only slightly more repeatable than the MCL. At this point the specialist merely converts the UCLs obtained in dB HL to dB SPL and prescribes them. However, there is no need for the amplifier to have an SSPL that exactly matches the client's UCL. Of course, it is undesirable for the SSPL to be higher than the UCLs, but as a minimum the louder speech sounds should go through the amplifier without undue clipping (Berger, 1980) (Berger, Hagberg & Rane, 1984). Thus, an output anywhere between the prescribed minimum and maximum is satisfactory.

To insure loud speech sounds not being unduly clipped we simply employ the operating gain (OG), which was previously determined, and to it add the level of loud speech at the four frequencies: 75dB at 500 Hz, 75 dB at 1000 Hz, 72 dB at 2000 Hz, and 70 dB at 4000 Hz. Where the hearing loss is not severe, and the unaided dynamic range not small, (we suggest no smaller than 35-40 dB) an SSPL anywhere between the computed minimum and maximum will be satisfactory. If the hearing loss is severe, and/or the dynamic range is small, the computed Minimum Desirable SSPL may be greater than the Maximum Permissible SSPL which, by definition, is incongruous. If the computed Minimum Desirable SSPL is close to the computed Maximum Permissible SSPL the clinician is alerted to potential problems of the hearing aid wearer. Specifically, soft speech sounds may not be adequately amplified or loud speech sounds may be undesirably clipped. If the average unaided dynamic range at 500 and 1000 Hz is smaller than about 35-40 dB, a compression amplifier of some variety is strongly indicated.

The predicted aided hearing threshold levels along with the two parts of the prescription might be written as follows for the 60 dB flat hearing loss example mentioned above. This is assuming UCLs for illustrative purposes to be 105 dB HL and the desired monaural fitting is for a behind-the-ear instrument for a sensorineural hearing loss:

	Maximum Gain	**Minimum Desirable SSPL**
500 Hz	40 dB	105 dB
1000 Hz	48 dB	(B)112 dB
2000 Hz	(A)52 dB	112 dB
3000 Hz	(A)48 dB	XX
4000 Hz	42 dB	102 dB
6000 Hz	40 dB	XX

(A) 2 dB added at 2000 Hz and 3 dB added at 3000 Hz for maximum gain only for behind-the-ear instruments as a 2cc coupler correction.

(B) Although minimum desirable SSPL at 1000 Hz calculates to 113 dB, it is limited to maximum permissible SSPL of 112 dB.

USING THE PRESCRIPTION

Having determined the two major components of our prescription (Maximum Gain at five or six frequencies, and Minimum Desirable and Maximum Permissible SSPL at four frequencies) the next step may now be taken. A hearing aid having maximum gain coming as close as possible to that given in the example above is desired. SSPL may be anywhere between the indicated Minimum Desirable SSPL and Maximum Permissible SSPL.

Using this generic prescription the specialist can search through technical data sheets to find the hearing aid model/setting most closely matching the prescription. Or, the prescription data can be sent to the manufacturer of choice with a request for a hearing aid approximating the prescribed factors. Obviously, there are thousands of possible prescription combinations, but only a limited number of amplifiers on the market. The chore is to find a hearing aid that most closely matches the desired prescriptive characteristics.

Another possibility is to use a computer to search for an appropriate hearing aid model/setting. In virtually all prescriptive methods a formula, or formulas, constitute the prescription. Formulas are particularly amenable to computerization. Thus, a small computer can be programmed to ask for the pertinent audiometric data (such as, thresholds, UCLs, air-bone gap), and then rapidly produce a generic prescription including desired aided thresholds. Advantages of the computer include the fact that it makes certain that you answer complete information, including some questions that might be overlooked (such as binaural vs. monaural fitting), and the generic prescription can be printed out so there is a permanent copy for the client's folder (Gans, Ver Hoef & Berger, 1983) (Berger, Gans & Ver Hoef, 1985).

With a slightly larger computer one can enter in assorted electroacoustic data from numerous hearing aids, either from one make or from assorted makes. In this case, one model may be entered several times if there is a tone control, earhook option, output control, etc. Once the computer has determined the generic prescription for a specific hearing loss case it can be used to search through entered data to find the model/setting coming closest to the prescription. Obviously, it takes a lot of time to enter the electroacoustic data, to add new instruments as they come out and delete instruments no longer available. But once this is done the computer can locate one or more hearing aids approximating the prescription much quicker and more accurately than can an individual by laboriously searching through technical data sheets. Hearing losses fall into a limited number of patterns (Berger, 1980) (Berger, 1980). Except for very mild and profound hearing losses there are ample hearing aid models available to approximate most prescriptions (Berger, Gans, 1986).

Some prescriptive procedures include not just the hearing aid make/model/setting but also other factors such as venting, tubing dimensions, and earmold horn effects. Our feeling is that any prescription is a first-order approximation of what is desired, and that individual differences in ear cavity dimensions, tympanic membrane stiffness, and perhaps other unknown individual differences affect the relationship between hearing loss and needed amplifier characteristics. Therefore, we use tone control changes, earhook alternatives, vent size changes, etc., as ways to alter the aided response if it differs from the predicted more than considered acceptable.

POST-FITTING TESTING

Once the client has been fitted with the prescribed hearing aid it is time to determine the effect of that amplification. To accomplish this it is desirable that the gain control of the hearing aid be set where the client usually has it. We place the client in the sound room, facing a loudspeaker (0 degree azimuth), and advise him to keep his nose pointed toward the loudspeaker and not to move the head. The client is instructed to respond to the discrete frequency signals (pulsing pure-tones, warbled tones, or narrow bands of noise, depending on the reflective characteristics of the walls in your sound room) as was done previously in the unaided condition. The same frequencies are tested as were prescribed for maximum gain. If there is any question of aided intolerance for loud sounds, the aided UCLs should also be determined.

We also routinely obtain aided SRT and word discrimination scores although, as previously noted, these are not an inherent part of the prescription. Aided word discrimination is tested at a 45 dB HL presentation.

From the aided test results, in comparison with those predicted, the specialist as well as the client can readily visualize how closely the aided response matches the predicted threshold. The difference between the unaided and aided thresholds constitutes functional gain. At this point, as noted above, minor alterations in the amplifier can be made if the aided response does not closely match that which was predicted. If there is a gross discrepancy between the predicted and aided responses, then an entirely new fitting effort is in order.

An advantage of determining the aided threshold with frequency specific stimuli is that by doing so changes in tone control settings, earmold modifications, possible later malfunction of the aid, etc., can be revealed. Word discrimination scores, or even speech reception thresholds, are not sensitive to such differentiations.

An alternative, or a supplement, to the aided sound field test is to use a probe tube technique. By comparing the unaided to aided probe tube response the equivalent of functional gain can be measured. An advantage of the probe tube technique is that a good sound treated room is not necessary, and no response is required of the client. It has also been assumed that the test-retest reliability of probe tube measures is a little better than that of functional gain measures.

Regardless of how the aided response is compared to the predicted (that is, prescribed) response, objectivity is added to the hearing aid fitting by making this comparison. Without such a comparison the specialist is left to rely on the comments and observations of the client, whose report may or may not be valid. Since clients most usually have been functioning with distorted hearing for a long period of time it seems unreasonable to expect them to make valid judgments about the appropriate frequency response or the correctness of the aided response. There is good evidence that it takes some time—days if not weeks—for most hearing aid wearers to adjust to and make best use of the new acoustic code presented by the amplifier. Logically, it is only after a period of adjustment to the hearing aid that either aided word discrimination scores or a listener's preference for a particular tone control setting have such meaningfulness.

ACCEPTANCE CRITERIA

Acceptance criteria for any hearing aid fitting are, at least at this time, arbitrary. Some would argue that if the client likes the hearing aid(s), or is satisfied with the aid(s), then this is an acceptable fitting. Liking a hearing aid, and being satisfied with it, seem related to the expectations of the client, degree and type of hearing loss, surely some personality factors, and no doubt to the person's social, vocational, and educational needs. Unfortunately, the dispenser has no test of "like" or "satisfaction," as much as we hope that the wearer likes the aid and is satisfied with it.

The logical acceptance criteria relate to the closeness of the obtained gain and SSPL to the prescribed gain and SSPL. That is, how closely was the goal reached? At the present time we are using an arbitrary acceptance criterion of ± 9 dB at 1000, 3000, and 4000 Hz, with a little larger permissible range for 6000 Hz. At 500 Hz we accept + 5 dB more gain than prescribed and − 9 dB; at 2000 Hz − 5 dB and + 9 dB. The reason for the slightly more stringent criteria at the latter two frequencies is that we don't want too much low-frequency sound going up the cochlea, so 5 dB is the most we accept at 500 Hz above that prescribed. As noted earlier 2000 Hz seems to be the most critical of all frequencies for speech understanding, so we don't accept a mismatch greater than 5 dB below that which was predicted. The specialist may, of course, set whatever acceptance criteria are desired. It is also of importance to make certain that the hearing aid wearer is not using the aid at full-on gain or at the lowest possible volume control setting. There should be some gain change possible in each direction, depending upon the user's typical wearing environments.

The prescriptive procedures outlined above do not specifically concern themselves with counselling the prospective hearing aid wearer or the person after being fitted. Suffice it to say that counselling and follow-up care are no less important with this than any other method.

RELIABILITY AND VALIDITY

In our judgment any person espousing a hearing aid fitting method of any kind should present the potential user of such a method with a rationale for what is to be done, and detailed procedures for accomplishing the method. In addition, the prospective user of a method deserves to have some published results available on successes and failures obtained with the method. A few "interesting cases" or a mere mean aided result from a small group of subjects does not give the prospective user adequate information on which to base a judgment about a given fitting method, whether it be prescriptive or not.

The professional literature, as might be expected, has produced little evidence on the subject of validity for any hearing aid fitting method, and not very much data for reliability. We can vouch for the difficulty in documenting either, in particular validity, although we have made a number of efforts to do so, which have been published (Berger, 1981) (Berger, Abel, Hagberg, La Puzz, Varavvas & Weldele, 1982) (Berger, Hagberg, 1982) (Berger, Varavvas, 1982) (Berger, Hagberg & Rane, 1984). A few independent studies have also involved the Berger Method (Bode, Cooper & Murray, 1980) (Nelson, Parker, 1982) (Hendler, 1987) and, in general, have found it acceptable if not excellent.

Only when a body of reliability and validity data are available on assorted hearing aid fitting protocols can we, as professionals, feel completely comfortable in choosing which method to routinely employ. Until then we are left open to criticisms and questions from outsiders about our fitting goals, methods, and results. Although much in hearing aid fitting still remains an "art" our goal should be to make it as much a science as is possible at any point in time. Prescription fittings, in my judgment, permit us to make a giant step toward that science, more so than other fitting methods, because they permit examining, microscopically, the prescription factors rather than a vague overall fitting result. Prescriptions permit ready computerization, and they all involve the use of numbers, in comparing what is needed to what was accomplished. Prescriptions place the decision as to what the electroacoustic characteristics should be upon the shoulders of the specialist, where it ought to be, rather than on the client or on some third party.

It is true that the precise electroacoustic factors needed for a given hearing loss are not known, but the prescription approaches have already begun to focus on the ideal little by little. Perhaps, because of individual differences and needs, we will never reach THE ideal, but certainly with prescriptive methods one can come much closer to the ideal than has been the case for the fitting methods used in the past.

SUMMARY

The rationale, procedures, and results for the Berger Method have been briefly outlined in this chapter, with the majority of space given to the first two subjects. However, all of these points, including considerable detail on results, have been published in readily accessible journals, monographs, and books. In the particular prescriptive method espoused in this chapter a maximum gain was prescribed at five or six frequencies, and SSPL was prescribed at four frequencies. Both were related to electroacoustic data obtained in a 2cc coupler, but modifications can quickly be made to relate the desired data to another coupler.

Once the electroacoustic characteristics have been prescribed a hearing aid approximating them is located and fitted to the client. The acceptance or rejection of the fitting is based upon how closely the obtained gain and SSPL match the predicted gain and SSPL. Where the mismatch between the predicted and obtained is small the dispenser can make changes in the earmold, tone control, tubing, etc., so as to more closely match the predicted. Where the obtained response is grossly different from that predicted an entirely new fitting effort is in order.

GLOSSARY

BSER Brain Stem Evoked Response. Electroencephalograph measures of brain-wave activity in response to a series of brief auditory signals, as recorded within 4 to 8 milliseconds of onset of the test signals.

COR Conditioned Orientation Reflex. A version of play audiometry which relies on the child's localizing ability as lighted stimuli are paired with sound coming from one of two loudspeakers.

Functional Gain The difference, in decibels, of sound measured with and without the hearing aid on an individual. Usually the measurement is done at the individual's threshold of sensitivity but may be accomplished at other levels.

Maximum Gain Full-on gain as measured with an input sound pressure level of 50 or 60 dB, as per ANSI-1976.

Maximum Permissible SSPL UCLs as measured in dB SPL or measured in dB HTL and converted to SPL.

Minimum Desirable SSPL Operating Gain at a given frequency plus the level of loud speech at that frequency.

Operating Gain Also called Preferred Gain or Use Gain. The amount of gain the hearing aid wearer chooses to employ under typical environmental conditions.

Reserve Gain Available gain above and beyond Operating Gain.

TROCA Tangible Reinforcement Operant Conditioning Audiometry. A type of audiometry wherein the child's correct responses to sound result in a small but tangible reward.

REFERENCES

The many published references to hearing aid fitting in general, or more specifically prescription fitting, may be found in the first chapter of this volume and in standard textbooks on the subject. It was considered appropriate here, despite possible charges of egotism, to list reports primarily related to this specific fitting method, in particular publications by the present author.

BERGER, K. W. The use of uncomfortable loudness level in hearing aid fitting. *Maico Audiological Library, Series,* 15:2, 1976.

BERGER, K. W. Prescription of hearing aids: a rationale. *Journal of the American Auditory Society,* 2, 1976, 71-78.

BERGER, K. W. The importance of the dynamic range in hearing aid fitting. *Zenetron Monographs,* 3, Nov. 1980.

BERGER, K. W. Threshold patterns in hearing aid fitting. *Hearing Journal,* 33:5, 1980, 4, 49.

BERGER, K. W. Gain requirements of identical audiograms. *Audiology & Hearing Education,* 6:1, 1980, 21, 29.

BERGER, K. W. Hearing aid selection and fitting by prescription. In Studies in the Use of Amplification (CI Berlin, ed.). *Excerpta Medica* for Zenetron, Inc., 1980, 29-43.

BERGER, K. W. Gain requirements of conductive hearing losses. *British Journal of Audiology,* 14, 1980, 137-141.

BERGER, K. W. Considerations of thresholds in fitting hearing aids. *Journal of Audiology Technique,* 20, 1981, 42-27.

BERGER, K. W. The reliability and validity of a hearing aid fitting method. *Hearing Journal,* 23:12, 1981, 6, 25-26.

BERGER, K. W. Is binaural for everyone? *Hearing Instruments,* 35:9, 1984, 24-26, 39.

BERGER, K. W., D. B. ABEL, E. N. HAGBERG, L. A. PUZZ, D. M. VARAVVAS, and F. J. WELDELE. Successes and problems of hearing aid users. *Hearing Journal,* 35:11, 1982, 26-30.

BERGER, K. W. and D. P. GANS. Matching electroacoustic responses to hearing loss patterns. *Audecibel,* 35:11, 1986, 16-18.

BERGER, K. W., D. P. GANS, and N. VERHOEF. Computerized hearing aid selection. *EHT Journal,* 85, 1985, 299-300.

BERGER, K. W. and E. N. HAGBERG. Gain usage based on hearing aid experience and subject age. *Ear & Hearing,* 3, 1982, 235-237.

BERGER, K. W. and E. N. HAGBERG. Hearing aid users report on hearing aid usage. *Monographs in Contemporary Audiology,* 3:4, Nov. 1982.

BERGER, K. W., E. N. HAGBERG, and R. L. RANE. One method of hearing aid prescription. *Hearing Instruments*, 29:7, 1978, 12-13.

BERGER, K. W., E. N. HAGBERG, and R. L. RANE. A prescriptive method of hearing aid fitting. *Audecibel*, 28, 1979, 32-40.

BERGER, K. W., E. N. HAGBERG, and R. L. RANE. Determining hearing aid gain. *Hearing Instruments*, 30:3, 1979, 26-28, 44.

BERGER, K. W., E. N. HAGBERG, and R. L. RANE. A re-examination of the one-half gain rule. *Ear & Hearing*, 1, 1980, 223-225. Reprinted in Audecibel, 30, 1981, 87-90.

BERGER, K. W., E. N. HAGBERG, and R. L. RANE. *Prescription Of Hearing Aids*. Kent, OH: Herald Publishing House, 4th ed. 1984.

BERGER, K. W., E. N. HAGBERG, D. M. VARAVVAS, and D. M. VOTTERO. Hearing threshold level and most comfortable loudness level in hearing aid prescription. *Ear & Hearing*, 3, 1982, 30-33.

BERGER, K. W., R. J. KLICH, and J. P. MILLIN. The speech spectrum in hearing aid fitting. *Audecibel*, 31:3, 1982, 18-20.

BERGER, K. W. and J. P. MILLIN. Choosing the binaural candidate and checking the fitting. In Binaural Hearing Aid Amplification (E. R. Libby, ed.), 1980, vol. 2.

BERGER, K. W., R. L. RANE, and E. N. HAGBERG. Comparisons of uncomfortable loudness levels and acoustic reflex thresholds. *Audiology & Hearing Education*, 5:2, 1979, 11-12, 14-15, 25.

BERGER, K. W. and L. L. SOLTISZ. Variability of thresholds and MCLs with speech babble. *Australian Journal of Audiology*, 3, 1981, 1-3.

BERGER, K. W. and D. M. VARAVVAS. Reliability in aided testing. *Hearing Journal*, 35, Feb. 1982, 7-9.

BERGER, K. W., D. M. VARAVVAS, and D. M. VOTTERO. Test-retest reliability of MCLs, UCLs, and ARTs with sensorineural loss subjects. *Hearing Instruments*, 35:5, 1982, 16, 19.

BODE, D. L., K. COOPER, and B. MURRAY. Selection of hearing aids for listeners with severe-profound impairment. A.S.H.A. convention presentation, Nov. 1980.

BROOKS, D. M. Gain requirements of hearing aid users. *Scandinavian Audiology*, 2, 1973, 199-205.

BYRNE, D. J. and D. FIFIELD. Evaluation of hearing aid fittings for infants. *British Journal of Audiology*, 8, 1974, 47-54.

CHRISTEN, R. and D. BYRNE. Variability of MCL measurements: significance for hearing aid selection. *Australian Journal of Audiology*, 2, 1980, 10-18.

DOMORACKI, D., K. W. BERGER, and J. P. MILLIN. A comparison of monaural and binaural gain settings. *Hearing Instruments*, 33:9, 1982, 18-19.

GANS, D. P., N. VERHOEF, and K. W. BERGER. Hearing aid selection by computer. *Hearing Instruments*, 34:5, 1983, 17, 97-98.

HENDLER, N. Evaluation of hearing aid fittings using Berger's method. *Audecibel*, 36:1, 1987, 22-24.

MARTIN, M.C. Hearing aid gain requirements in sensorineural hearing loss. *British Journal of Audiology*, 7, 1973, 21-24.

McCANDLESS, G. A. and D. L. MILLER. Loudness discomfort and hearing aids. *Hearing Journal*, 25:8, 1972, 7, 28, 32.

MILLIN, J. P. Speech discrimination as a function of hearing-aid gain: implications in hearing-aid evaluation. MA thesis, Western Reserve University, 1965.

MORRIS, T. An approach to calculating gain requirements for severely deaf children as a function of hearing loss which is independent of frequency response. *Scandinavian Audiology*, 6, 1977, 21-25.

NELSON, P. B. and R. M. PARKER. A comparison of traditional vs. formula hearing aid selection procedures using probe microphones. A.S.H.A. convention presentation, Nov. 1982.

SHORE, I., R. C. BILGER, and I. J. HIRSH. Hearing aid evaluation: reliability of repeated measurements. *J. Speech Hearing Disorders*, 25, 1960, 152-170.

IV

POGO METHOD OF HEARING AID SELECTION

GEARY A. McCANDLESS

INTRODUCTION

Hearing impairment is characterized primarily by a loss of sensitivity or acuity. Restoration of loss of functional acuity is achieved by amplifying sound to the pathologic ear. We know that impaired ears, especially sensorineural disorders, have numerous functional changes other than that of reduced sensitivity, such as greater loss in some frequencies than others, reduction of the dynamic range, and various types of internal distortion. Hearing aids in no way alter or improve the inherent characteristics of the pathologic ear nor improve actual thresholds. They only improve functional acuity by making sound louder. Even with the novel approaches to signal processing we cannot yet compensate for the distortion in the pathologic ear. We can through a hearing aid, make sound louder and emphasize frequency bands having greatest loss. We can also limit loud sounds to a comfortable listening level, making communication and hearing environmental sound possible for individuals with impaired hearing.

It is reasonable to assume that for any one hearing loss, a given range of electroacoustic characteristics will provide an optimum in speech intelligibility and subjective pleasantness of sound quality. Recent studies strongly indicate that when a hearing aid provides optimum speech intelligibility it also is judged by the user as being pleasant in sound quality (Byrne and Dillon, 1986). This implies that if the proper electroacoustic characteristic can be specified for good speech intelligibility it will be well accepted by the user in terms of sound quality. Further, it argues for the notion of prescribing or specifying optimum electroacoustic requirements for hearing aid users since a prescription provides a good or fitting objective from which to design and provide a hearing aid.

It should be stressed here, that a prescriptive or predictive procedure does not disregard the fact that acoustic requirements vary with each hearing loss, nor is it suggested that a prescriptive fitting properly completed may not require final "tweaking" or tuning to optimize intelligibility, quality, or other requirements of a specific patient. A prescriptive approach does, however, imply that if based on a sound rationale, and if the specific characteristics are achieved, it provides, in an efficient way, a close approximation of the need of the user.

Prescriptive fitting also has the advantage of being both valid and rapidly done. This improves the cost effectiveness in a clinic or busy office while not sacrificing clinical quality.

A second point of importance must be made here. Fitting aids by prescription has an objective of providing or introducing certain acoustic properties to a pathologic ear which will maximally compensate for specific auditory deficiencies. Its greatest value, therefore, lies in setting a goal or clear fitting objective in terms of gain/frequency response and maximum output, which if met in the actual hearing aid hardware, provides a close approximation of the final aid, mold and tubing.

Calculating a hearing aid prescription is but the first in several fitting steps. The prescription specifies the gain and output which, if provided, should yield improved measured speech intelligibility scores and good subjective quality. Following calculation, a good fitting procedure must implement the prescription by translating desired characteristics into actual hardware. This is done by selection and adjustment of molds, tubing, and stock aids, or by the manufacturers who by their own prescription, provide a so called "customized" aid. Finally, after determination of desired characteristics and selection of an aid, the goals of the prescription must be verified by measurement, otherwise there is no way of knowing whether or not optimum gain and output requirements have been met. Verification may also include speech intelligibility or subjective listening tests. The prescription merely provides the gain, power and response requirements from which the fitter/clinician can make any final adjustments to maximize the comfort and clarity of the aid.

RATIONALE FOR THE POGO FITTING PROCEDURE

There is consensus among professionals that some type of selection procedure is desirable; that differing frequency response and output levels are required for different hearing losses. However, there is poor agreement as to what specific acoustic requirements are best or whether general characteristics over a broad range are adequate for most hearing impairments. It is believed by some that one or two frequency responses are appropriate for all degrees and shapes of hearing loss (Davis, et al, 1947). Others question the merit of an evaluation or selection at all. The most widely used fitting technique over the last forty years was one proposed by Carhart (1946) who made a selection from a number of stock aids. Selections were made based on the lowest aided threshold and highest speech discrimination scores. The wide-spread use of this procedure persists today even though it is very time consuming and shows poor reliability (Shore, Bilger, and Hirsh, 1960). More important, such comparative techniques based solely on speech scores do not identify which of the electroacoustic characteristics contribute or detract from the speech recognition results. Such selection techniques preclude identifying which parameters should be altered to improve speech function or subjective quality. Selection of aids by speech scores in general does not assist in making frequency response/ gain adjustments, they merely reflect which aid or setting of an aid yields the best scores, provided the resultant speech score differences are sufficiently large.

Fitting by so called prescription is not new. In fact advance calculation of specific gain requirement was found among the earliest fitting procedures beginning about 1930. One reason fitting by prescription did not become more popular was that neither adequate clinical nor research data were available upon which to establish ideal characteristics to the pathologic ear. Further, the relationship between a properly fitted auditory prescription and subject satisfaction was not clearly established. A prescriptive or other procedure succeeds only in as far as it results in improved aided function and an acceptable level of satisfaction from the user. There is no reason to carefully prescribe specific acoustic properties for a hearing aid nor to select an aid other than by subjective quality judgement of ''satisfactory'' unless the resultant fitted aid yields improved function. Recent research gives impressive evidence that fitting by prescription does in fact result in high patient satisfaction and also optimizes speech intelligibility (Byrne and Dillon, 1986). It is reasonable that compensating for the specific deficiencies found in each individual hearing loss will potentially yield best aided hearing. Further, most prescriptive techniques, including POGO, assume that if accurate and most significant psychoacoustic (audiometric) measures are obtained and appropriately translated into a hearing aid, high speech recognition and satisfaction will occur (McCandless and Lyregaard, 1983). The POGO technique also assumes that measures other than speech stimuli, i.e., pure tone or narrow band noise, are best used to specify required gain and output. After initial fitting, speech discrimination or a qualitative test can then be used if desired for final verification of fit.

Basic to any prescriptive method is the rationale upon which it is based. Current prescriptive techniques reflect basic philosophies regarding the restoration of function to the pathologic ear. Some differing rationales or objectives for prescriptive fitting are summarized as follows:

> To provide gain appropriate to achieve functional threshold shifts towards normal hearing (Berger, 1977).
>
> To present the average speech spectrum at a comfortable level to the ear (Berger, 1976; Pascoe, 1975; Byrne and Tonisson, 1976; Watson and Knudsen, 1940).
>
> To provide maximum dynamic intensity range to the ear.
>
> To provide equal aided hearing levels to the ear (Pascoe, 1975).
>
> To provide aided signals that restore equal loudness function (Victoreen, 1973; Wallenfels, 1967).
>
> To provide aided speech signals at the most comfortable listening levels in the speech frequencies (Pascoe, 1975; Shapiro, 1976; Bragg, 1977).
>
> Provide gain based on the size and shape of the dynamic range (Wallenfels, 1976; Kee, 1972).

Prescriptive techniques hold promise as the method of choice for hearing aid evaluation since specific auditory deficits can be quantified by test and measurable electroacoustic characteristics can be calculated and provided (minimally, gain and output). Despite the differences underlying the basic philosophies in prescription methods they appeared to contain some basic similarities. The major limitations in current prescriptive techniques appeared to be: (1) Lack of clear rationale for specifying optimum or ''best'' gain, and SSPL for specific hearing losses; (2) Absence of techniques for accurately translating desired characteristics into wearable hearing aids; (3) The lack of objective clinical criteria to validate the prescription with real-ear measures.

CHAPTER OBJECTIVES

The basic goals of POGO fitting procedure were to derive a method which combines simplicity with practicality which results in optimum aided speech intelligibility and qualitative sound pleasantness.

Although this procedure is designed to fit a *particular* ear, it applies appropriately to binaural and other special fitting requirements. Application of the process is simple though the derivation of the formula and fitting steps was complex. The procedure is intended to provide a close approximation of required characteristics, which in the authors experience, and by research evidence, will constitute a near-best possible choice of electroacoustic values for current hearing aids. In practice it provides an efficient way to arrive at a starting point, or close approximation, from which subsequent fine adjustments can be made as required by the user. Implicit, too, is the plan for adjustment and upgrading of the procedure as technology provides new sound processing schemes or whenever evidence indicates the need for change.

Basic requirements in development of the POGO procedure were:

1 It must be efficient and capable of administration within the time constraints of a busy office or clinic.

2 It must yield a fitting which has acceptable sound quality to the user, yet optimize speech intelligibility in a wide variety of environmental settings.

3 It should be scientifically sound with a strong rationale for each step or routine used.

4 It should require a minimum of specialized equipment (although some is essential) and be capable of administration in a sound treated (not anechoic) environment.

5 As far as possible, it should be applicable to most ages and to special populations, thus selective tests which require difficult subjective quality judgements are not appropriate because of their inherent variability.

The POGO procedure arose because existing procedures merely specified desired characteristics, or just measured function, but lacked specifics as to how to arrive at a proper fitting. The POGO procedure was developed to provide a complete, efficient, and comprehensive method of selection, implementation, and verification of the fit. Stated differently, POGO (1) specifies the acoustic requirements for individual patients; (2) provides a technique for translating these requirements into a wearable hearing aid; and (3) provides a method of verification of fit with the earmold and tubing in place and produces "optimum" hearing and evidence of qualitative pleasantness. It is felt by the author that procedures lacking all three steps are incomplete and compromise clinical effectiveness. Certainly any predictive or prescriptive technique must have a verification procedure to assess whether or not the prescriptive goals have been met.

The POGO fitting method is designed primarily for sensory (cochlear) losses, and for conductive losses with proper computational corrections. The basic formula is applied to sensory losses only and is best applied to losses less than about 90 dB. The method at present does not attempt to define whether or not a hearing aid is to be recommended, nor which ear to fit, or if binaural aids are appropriate. It is relevant only in providing a correctly shaped amplified signal to the pathologic ear and specified upper limit of amplification. The formula at present applies to hearing aids with linear amplifier or with aids using compression primarily to limit intense sound. This should *not* be interpreted to mean that aids with compression capability are inappropriate for use with POGO. In fact, virtually all hearing aids available today utilize linear amplifiers. In normal use they operate on the linear portion of the gain curve. Compression is used as a form of output limiting and is rarely used to reduce a wide intensity range to a narrow dynamic hearing range. Current compression aids are almost always used merely as a method of protecting the user from intense sound by limiting the output to acceptable loudness levels.

ONE HALF GAIN RULE

The principles under the POGO procedure are based on the fact that a sensory loss is accompanied by recruitment making sounds of low or moderate intensity inordinately weak, whereas intense sounds are as loud as they would be for normal hearing persons. Conventional amplifiers (linear) amplify both weak and intense sounds equally, often making louder environmental sounds intolerable and soft sounds inaudible to the recruiting ear. The solution at present is to compromise the optimum amount of gain in order to keep other sounds within a comfortable range. Gain calculations are made such that sounds most important in line are placed near the most comfortable loudness level. Practical experience as well as theoretical considerations, indicate a good gain goal is the half gain principle where optimum insertion gain is equal to about one half the hearing loss. This general formula was first proposed by Lybarger (1963), and when applied to hearing aid use, provides sufficient gain for mild and moderate losses to hear most speech at conversational levels.

Hearing losses amenable to hearing aid use have three major characteristics:

1 A loss of sensitivity (hearing loss) often unequal at various frequencies.

2 An individual upper intensity limit or discomfort threshold, above which the patient will not tolerate, if exposed over time.

3 Cochlear losses which constitute more than 95% of hearing aid candidates, show a narrowing of the dynamic range caused not by

reduction of tolerance levels, but by a reduction of the hearing range between the threshold of acuity and threshold of discomfort.

To compensate for the auditory deficits above, selection of two of the three (gain and output) electroacoustic characteristics are essential. At present the POGO formula does not include the type nor amount of compression, since compression acts largely to protect the ear and not to compress the total intensity range to fit the subject dynamic range. Further, there are many types and applications of compression, the effects of which are not well understood or predictable.

Even with the novel approaches to electroacoustic modification or exotic signal processing, we cannot yet compensate for the distortion found in the pathologic ear. Virtually all prescriptive procedures specify required gain/frequency response goals for the hearing aid candidate and a few, including POGO, specify maximum output levels. Although the electroacoustic properties describing hearing aids, gain and output are the parameters most often used for formulae, two parameters are intended to compensate for specific psychoacoustic requirements in the ear: compensation of loss of acuity (gain) and second, to limit the amplified sounds to levels which do not overload the system and become uncomfortable (SSPL). Compression in most current hearing aids serve only to protect the user from intense sound but does not truly compensate for a narrow dynamic range through a non linear amplifying system. The characteristics of a pathologic ear and the acoustic characteristics used to compensate for these deficits are:

Characteristic of Hearing Deficit	Electroacoustic Characteristic Used to Compensate or Control
1. Loss of sensitivity at various frequencies.	Shaping the gain/frequency response.
2. Threshold of discomfort.	Saturation sound pressure limiting or other output limiting.
3. Narrow dynamic range.	Certain types and characteristics of compression.

DERIVATION OF POGO GAIN/FREQUENCY

Even though the POGO calculation of ideal insertion gain is based on threshold values, the resultant gain does shift speech and other sounds correctly into the patients most comfortable listening range (MCL). This shift into the MCL range is actually controlled by the user's volume control. Use of hearing threshold level (HTL) to calculate gain is utilized for convenience without the necessity of measuring patient's own MCL, a measure which is variable, time consuming, and obtained with great difficulty for most potential hearing aid users. Further, it cannot be used for children nor for special populations since they cannot give valid MCL measures.

The actual POGO gain/output formula was developed from a series of studies designed to carefully define the optimum listening levels for various degrees and types of hearing impairment. Optimum frequency response characteristics were further specified based on speech intelligibility tests, and subjective measures of overall pleasantness of sound quality, from 200 hearing aid users. Values constituting the final gain formula were developed by analyzing over 40 prescriptive formulae. Detailed analyses compared the gain requirements from eight procedures used successfully and provided a reasonable rationale for their use. The gain requirement for various hearing impairments for the eight procedures were then averaged as illustrated for one hearing loss as shown in Figure 1. The intent was to measure which technique had the least cumulative deviation from the mean gain values, and from the mean value determine through the clinical efficacy and subject satisfaction through clinical studies. Clinic results do indeed indicate that fitting according to the POGO formula results in good user benefit and

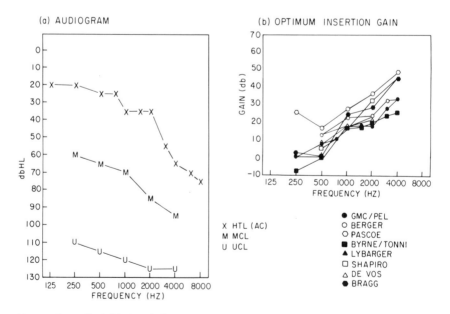

Fig. 1. Prescribed ideal gain/frequency characteristics calculated from eight different procedures for a typical, mild, high frequency sensorineural hearing loss.

acceptance. From the procedures above, the POGO gain/frequency response formula evolved as follows:

Frequency	Insertion Gain (dB)
250	1/2 HTL — 10
500	1/2 HTL — 5
1000	1/2 HTL
2000	1/2 HTL
3000	1/2 HTL
4000	1/2 HTL

Note: For conductive losses, insertion gain should equal the amount of loss but add the low frequency cut of −10 dB at 250 Hz and −5 dB at 500 Hz.

DERIVATION OF MAXIMUM OUTPUT USING THE POGO FORMULA

Of the two parameter specifications used in the formula, i.e., gain and output, limiting output to proper levels is often a greater determinant of success than other factors. The necessity of setting proper output cannot be overstressed. More hearing aid dissatisfaction and rejection results not from excessive gain (as this can be adjusted by the volume control), but from SSPL levels which are too high. It can be stated without reservation, that most current hearing aids available today have excessive output well above the tolerable levels in the pathologic ear. Users attempt to compensate for excessive output by reducing the hearing aid gain which in fact only makes function poorer, as lowering the volume also makes softer sounds inaudible.

The second electroacoustic parameter used in POGO is that of output. The inclusion of frequency response in a formula specified only the spectral shape of the signals to be delivered to the ear, but ignores the requirement to limit output to a safe, comfortable level.

Deciding appropriate output was complicated by the lack of consensus as to what this level should be for a given patient. Some clinicians believe output should be high to prevent distortion and that the user must learn to adjust to intense sounds or "toughen" the ear. Others, including this author, believe output must be limited to a point of *beginning* discomfort since long term sound above this level will not be acceptable to the user. Further, it assumes that basically most sound must be in a comfort or MCL range with an aid, just as it is for normally hearing subjects. The rationale for POGO goes even further: A hearing aid which presents sound at levels proportionally higher than to which the normal ear is exposed, is either poorly engineered, improperly fit or both.

Arriving at optimum output levels requires specific measurement of loudness overload or discomfort, translation of these measures correctly into a hearing aid then final subject verification that the aid does not produce unacceptably loud sounds. This presupposes that psychoacoustic (threshold of discomfort) measures are made for each subject in HL and translated to the aid to be used (in SPL).

For the final formula, calculation of optimum output, a series of studies were done to determine what instructions, stimuli and measures seemed most appropriate, practical and valid for clinical use. Early in these studies it became clear that instructions for determining discomfort levels greatly influence the so-called "tolerance" level. Reports from other investigators as to average tolerance levels were highly variable, depending on the stimuli and instructions used (McCandless, G. A., 1978).

To better define, for formula fitting purposes, what constitutes an upper loudness limit for hearing aids, the author conducted a series of studies to explore discomfort or overload as specifically related to a wearable aid. Results of these studies showed:

1   A measured discomfort level can be influenced up to about 20 dB by the instructions used in obtaining that measure.

2   The majority (over 65%) of hearing aid users complained of loudness discomfort with their aid, indicating excessive SSPL.

3   Contrary to the common notion that the UCL is a psychological parameter or measure, research clearly shows that physiological (autonomic nervous system) responses appear at or near a point judged to be *beginning* discomfort. This suggests physiological as well as psychological loudness overload.

4   That aids whose output were limited to the patient's threshold or beginning discomfort levels consistently produced more acceptable and successfully fitted aids.

5   The appropriate clinical instructions for discomfort for hearing aid application is *threshold* of discomfort. Instruction using words as "too loud," intolerably loud, distinctively uncomfortable, or too loud to listen to for 15 minutes, tend to produce discomfort measures which, if translated to hearing aids, are too loud for long time use.

6   The upper usable levels or levels at which hearing aids should be limited for sensory losses is *lower* than previously thought. Figure 2 shows the average threshold of discomfort (UCL) for 64 subjects with sensory loss. There is about a 20 dB upward shift in the discomfort threshold (UCL) for a 100 dB shift in hearing loss.

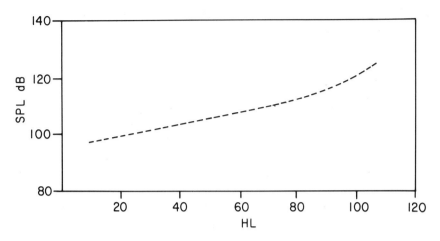

Fig. 2. Average uncomfortable loudness thresholds in dB HL for sixty-four subjects with losses from 10 to 100 dB.

The formula used for POGO calculation specifying *peak* output is equal to the average UCL in dB HL measured with earphones at 500, 1000, and 2000 Hz. To convert this average UCL SPL for selection of a hearing aid, add 4 dB:

$$\text{Desired individual SSPL} = \frac{\text{UCL 500} + \text{UCL 1000} + \text{UCL 2000} + 4}{3}$$

USING THE POGO METHOD

As previously stated, the prescription of gain/output (POGO) contains three basic steps: Step 1: *Calculation* of the desired or required characteristics — gain and output based on audiometric pure tone thresholds and pure tone thresholds of discomfort. Step 2: *Implementation* translation of the required gain and SSPL into an actual hearing aid including all tubing, molds, and other acoustic modifications. Step 3: *Verification* of acoustical performance. This step implies measurement of the two prescribed parameters: gain/frequency response and output. This step assures that the objectives in step one have been achieved. This portion of the procedure step is essential due to the large intersubject variations of acoustical performance of the aid and earmolds to be adequately modified. Most importantly, tangible evidence of performance can be quickly and validly quantified.

AUDIOMETRIC MEASURES AND CALCULATION OF DESIRED GAIN/ FREQUENCY RESPONSE

Conventional audiometric pure tone and threshold of discomfort levels are first made as shown in the example in Figure 3. Calculation of the required *insertion,* or effective gain values are then plotted on the gain chart as shown. Desired insertion gain or predicted aided thresholds can also be noted on the audiogram form to illustrate the projected aided threshold levels. The insertion gain on the audiogram is used both for purposes of illustration and for later verification measurement of the aided versus unaided thresholds with a final selected aid set at a comfort level setting. The required insertion gain curve chart represents desired insertion gain in dB delivered by the patient's hearing aid set at a comfortable level, and serves as the basis for choosing the gain for specific aids.

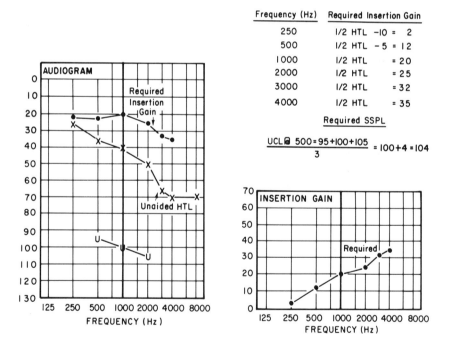

Fig. 3. Audiometric test results, and calculated desired insertion gain and desired output for a subject with a mild sensorineural hearing loss.

Also shown in Figure 3 is the peak SSPL level, in this case 104 dB SPL, which is the maximum output measured in a 2cc coupler to which the aid must be limited.

To summarize this step:

1 Obtain pure tone thresholds.

2 Obtain UCL measures at 500, 1000, and 2000 Hz.

3 Plot desired insertion gain on chart and on audiogram.

4 Calculate required SSPL.

IMPLEMENTATION

The objective of this step is to find which of the hearing aids or characteristics of aids best fit the ideal gain and output requirements. This assumes, of course, that the selections are being made from clinic aids in stock or from manufacturers specification sheets. For so-called "custom" fitting, especially of ITE aids, implementation selection of desired characteristics is, in fact, made by the manufacturers using their own prescriptive projections. The prescriptive fitting criteria for each manufacturer is not usually known, therefore, it is recommended that specific gain/output requirements be specified at time of the evaluation and sent to the manufacturer. Desired gain and output characteristics are best expressed in insertion gain plus reserve or full on gain 2cc coupler gain values.

In practice, the goal is to quickly and efficiently select an appropriate aid, including modifications which will most nearly meet the previously calculated requirements. First, determine if the required SSPL is within the adjustment range of the aid. Using the example in Figure 3 the peak SSPL should not exceed 104 dB. Second, find an aid with peak gain in the 500-2000 Hz range and check to determine if the shape is appropriate and that 10 dB reserve gain is provided. Keep in mind the range of gain and output adjustment for each aid. Remember that internal gain adjustments and output controls are rarely independent. This means that when the output is adjusted, the gain is also affected and vice versa.

In selecting proper aid characteristics also keep in mind that for the purposes of fitting, you are looking for an aid meeting the calculated requirements. These calculations are SSPL as measured at 2cc coupler and frequency response (insertion gain) and made as if the aid were on the user set at a comfortable level at less than full volume. Stated differently, we are trying to fit a desired insertion gain curve yet most manufacturers give electroacoustic data as measured in 2cc couplers at

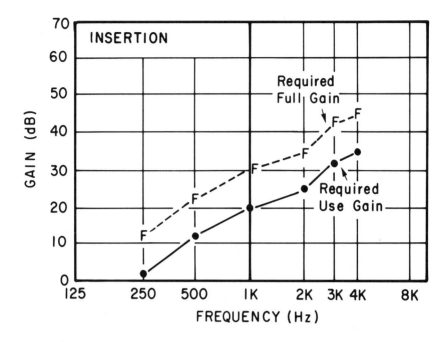

Fig. 4. Required insertion gain requirements at a comfort level setting, plus a desired or calculated full gain curve. This upper curve is derived simply by adding 10 dB (reserve gain) to the desired insertion gain curve.

full volume. Some manufacturers do list characteristics of aids as measured on the KEMAR® manikin or Zwislocki coupler at a reference test gain setting. These differences in format must be kept in mind in selecting an aid having the proper characteristics.

If insertion gain data are not available, selection can be accomplished using full-on-gain 2cc coupler data available from most manufacturers. The following technique for rapid pre-selection is useful: Using the required insertion gain curve previously plotted for the hearing aid candidate, draw a curve 10 dB above the desired insertion curve as shown in Figure 4. This curve is the required gain (at a comfort level setting) plus reserve (10 dB) equally, a proper aid as if set at *full volume.* This new desired full gain curve can be used for direct comparisons of manufacturers' data also expressed in full gain configuration. Drawing the curve takes only a few seconds but permits direct translation of manufacturers' data to the needs of the patient. The only other consideration being that 2cc coupler data over-estimates what is typically found at the ear, and must be corrected as shown in the following table.

| | Frequency | | | | | |
Type of Aid	200	500	1000	2000	3000	4000
ITE	3	1	2	−6	−6	5
BTE	3	1	0	−2	−11	−9
Body	3	7	10	−11	−13	−13

Actual number will depend somewhat on microphone position, shape of the aid, etc. Also canal aids provide greater inherent gain above 2000 Hz than other ITE devices so less correction can be made.

Figure 5 illustrates the desired gain curve, desired full on gain curve as well as a typical ITE hearing aid frequency response curve at full volume from the manufacturer. Note that the 2cc coupler gain seems excessive, but after subtracting the correction factor, this aid is quite appropriate for fitting and verification steps.

When ordering an aid from the manufacturer, this technique can be used to request appropriate gain and output. It is valuable in that the clinician assumes the responsibility for the desired characteristics for his patient's hearing aid. Further, there is greater likelihood the desired characteristics will be provided to the patient's ear.

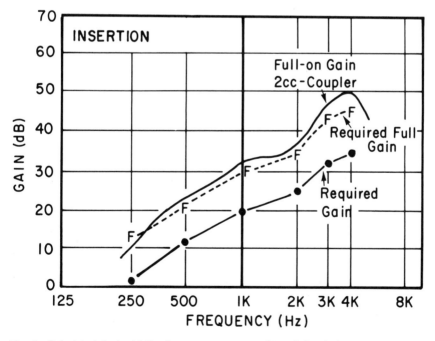

Fig. 5. Calculated desired full gain curve as compared to a full gain frequency response curve of a typical hearing aid measured in a 2cc coupler.

POGO PROCEDURE AND ACOUSTIC MODIFICATIONS

The basic POGO formula calculations are based on fitting using a closed earmold with a standard bore. However, the desired gain and output requirements apply as a goal or fitting objective no matter what aid or acoustic modification is used. For example, once the desired calculations are made, it matters little whether the criteria are met using a closed or open mold, or whether output control is made by internal adjustment or by venting. What is important is that the predicted frequency response/gain values are adequately shaped and supplied and that output is limited to coincide with the upper usable limits of the patient.

In selecting an aid or implementing the formula calculation, one must include the expected modifications produced by venting, open molds, horn and filter effects. These modifications must be included and applied to each potential hearing aid. In general, venting cuts low frequencies below 500 Hz; opening the earmold cuts frequencies below 2000 Hz; an open mold fitting may cut output at all frequencies, and a horn effect tends to augment frequencies above 2000 Hz. These modifications are illustrated in Figure 6. As applied to POGO simply add or subtract these modifications to the closed mold specifications. Because of the variations caused by interactions of canal size and shape and other factors, acoustic modifications cannot be precisely predicted; therefore, their effects should be estimated, and the verification of their effects must be made using insertion gain measures.

VERIFICATION OF FIT

The whole notion of prescribing or predicting desired acoustic characteristics presupposes that the goals can be met. Calculation of desired characteristics and selection of an aid provides an approximation of ideal gain/output but in no way guarantees these parameters are deliv-

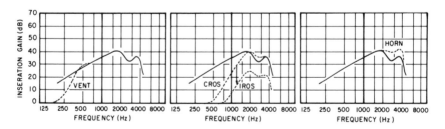

Fig. 6. Typical effects of venting, open molds, and horns on the frequency response curve.

ered in the actual fitting. Source of variations difficult to predict are: canal size and volume, microphone position, size and location of vents, size of mold opening, size and position of horn gain and output characteristics, impedance of the client's auditory system.

The use of POGO or other predictive formula necessitates a verification that the objectives have been met — else why bother to calculate fitting goals at all. The use of POGO implies that a subject's requirements are first determined by psychoacoustic (audiometric) testing. The target, desired characteristic, or requirement are calculated. Implicit in this rationale is the notion that target requirements can be translated into an actual hearing aid including tubing and earmolds. Also it is assumed that the criteria are closely adhered to, so the user will derive adequate or optimum benefit and satisfaction.

Verification as used in POGO is the process of measuring or quantifying insertion or functional gain when the aid is on the patient and volume set at a comfortable level.

VERIFYING GAIN/FREQUENCY RESPONSE

Verification must be checked in situ, i.e., on the ear wearing the hearing aid. Two techniques are used for verification that gain is proper, each of which is acceptable. The first is functional insertion gain. The test is performed by measuring the aided sound field thresholds for warble tones or narrow band noise. If testing equipment is calibrated in HL, the aided results can be compared with thresholds under phones. When the sound field is uncalibrated, functional insertion gain is the difference in thresholds or improvement in dB of aided versus unaided. It is recommended these measures be performed at 1 meter distance at 0° azimuth taking care to occlude or mask the opposite ear if necessary. The second verification procedure is insertion gain measured with one of several probe microphone devices. The characteristics of the subject's ear are measured first, then compared with those when the aid is in place and turned on. This resultant insertion gain can then be compared with the previously calculated ideal insertion gain curve plotted as shown in Figure 7. As a general rule, the measured gain curve should not deviate more than 5 dB from the target curve at any frequency from 250-4000 Hz.

VERIFYING SSPL

This process is to see that the SSPL does not permit sounds through the hearing aid to exceed the patient's UCL. This is essentially a functional output check using the patient's own sensation of "too loud" to set the

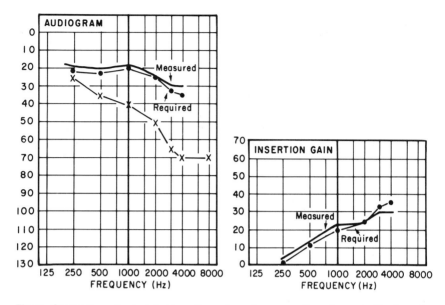

Fig. 7. Comparison of calculated insertion gain and measured insertion gain. The insertion gain can be subtracted from the pure tone thresholds and plotted on the audiogram as also shown, or can be directly measured in sound field or by probe insertion measurement.

upper usable output limit. The test is performed by turning the volume control to full. In a sound field, gradually turn up a narrow band noise (NBN) or warble tone to 80 dB HL. If this can be done without reaching the patient's UCL, the SSPL setting is considered satisfactory. If not, the output of the aid must be considered inappropriate. An alternate procedure is to present speech live voice directed at the aid or via a speaker system at a level of 80 dB SPL and check for discomfort.

FINAL ADJUSTMENT AND SUBJECTIVE VERIFICATION

It may happen that the hearing aid may fail to match the required characteristics. In such a case, the aid, mold or other adjustments must be made to better meet the desired acoustic goals. At this point, a careful comparison between the ideal and measured data are helpful as a guide to whatever modification may be required.

Subjective verification should also be a part of final verification. While the new acoustic pattern may sound strange, especially to new users, the quality should not be unpleasant. In fact, there is an excellent reported correlation between measured intelligibility and subjective pleasantness. In rare cases slight modifications may be required to satisfy the impressions of the user, being careful not to compromise gain in frequency bands which can compromise speech intelligibility.

SUMMARY

The POGO technique was designed to provide a simple, rapid and practical method of optimizing the electroacoustic characteristics for a given hearing loss. It represents a consensus of several successful existing procedures, plus basic research data relative to the acoustic requirements of the pathologic ear. Not only is the procedure simple and produces a high ratio of successful well accepted fittings, but it can be performed in a very short time. After conventional audiometric testing, calculations of ideal characteristics can be completed in less than one minute. Implementation or selection of a specific aid or set of characteristics to be ordered from the manufacturer require but a few minutes. Verification, too, requires either aided puretones and tolerance measures, or insertion gain measures, both procedures taking five or six minutes.

In the final analysis, the user must live with the aid. Fitting by the POGO procedure provides an aid most likely to be well liked by the patient. Through fast efficient aid selection, the clinician can spend adequate time in orientation, counselling, and possible minor ''tweaking'' of the aid. This is sometimes neglected due to constraints of time.

GLOSSARY

Comparative fitting technique A hearing aid selection procedure where a ''best'' or ''optimum'' aid or characteristics of aids are selected among stock aids or specifications. Criteria for superior performance are usually speech thresholds and discrimination scores.

Desired (Ideal) electroacoustic characteristics: The characteristics of a hearing aid, usually gain/frequency response, output or others, considered optimal for the hearing loss of a specific patient. These characteristics are thought to produce best or highly satisfactory function as well as probable subjective pleasantness.

Desired full-gain curve: Using the POGO formula, this is the calculated frequency response/gain curve determined by adding ten dB (reserve gain) to the ideal insertion gain curve. This calculated full-gain curve permits fairly direct comparison with manufacturer's published full gain frequency response curves.

Desired (Ideal) insertion gain: Using POGO or other predictive formula, a frequency response/gain curve is calculated which represents the desired or target functional difference (improvement) between unaided and aided thresholds over a normal frequency range.

Desired (Ideal) SSPL: The maximum peak or average output to be integrated into an individual's hearing aid as calculated by POGO or other predictive formula.

Hearing aid formula or prescription: A calculation of the desired frequency response/gain, SSPL, or other characteristics to be achieved in a wearable hearing aid for a specific hearing aid candidate.

Insertion gain: The difference in gain/frequency response referenced at the eardrum, measured with a functioning hearing aid in place and without the hearing aid. Currently, insertion gain is measured with probe tubes placed in the external ear canal.

POGO: Prescription Of Gain and Output. A predictive hearing aid fitting technique which includes procedures for calculating: (1) ideal gain and output; (2) implementing the characteristics into actual hearing aids; and (3) methods of verifying that target criteria of gain and output have been achieved.

Threshold of discomfort: The intensity at which a sound stimulus is perceived as beginning to be uncomfortably loud. This is contrasted with discomfort measures which require the stimulus to be "clearly" uncomfortable, intolerable, or louder than they would like to listen to for a period of time.

REFERENCES

BERGER, K. W. (1976). *Prescription of hearing aids: A rationale.* Kent State University.

BRAGG, V. C. (1977). Toward more objective hearing aid fitting procedures. *Hearing Instruments, 28* (9), 6-9.

BYRNE, P., & TONISSON, W. (1976). Selecting the gain of hearing aids for persons with sensorineural hearing impairments. *Scand. Audio, 5,* 51-59.

BYRNE, D., & DILLON, H. L. (1986). The national acoustic laboratories (NAL) new procedure for selecting the gain and frequency response of a hearing aid. *Ear and Hearing, 7* (4), 257-265.

CARHART, R. (1946). Selection of hearing aids. *Arch. Otolaryngology, 44,* 1-18.

DAVIS, H., STEVEN, S. S., NICHOLAS, R. H., JR., HUDGINS, C. V., MARQUIS, R. J., PERSON, E. G., & ROSS, D. A. (1947). Hearing aids: Experimental study of design objectives. Cambridge, MA: Harvard University Press.

KEE, W. R. (1972). Use of pure tone measurement in hearing aid fittings. *Audecibel,* 19-15.

LYBARGER, S. F. (1963). *Simplified fitting system for hearing aids.* Radioear Specifications and Fitting Information Manual, 1-8.

McCANDLESS, G. A., & LYREGAARD, P. E. (1983). Prescription of gain/output for hearing aids. *Hearing Instruments, 34* (8), 16-21.

McCANDLESS, G. A. (1978, February). *Critical factors in hearing aid fitting.* Proceedings of the Second International Conference Audiology Technology. Alexander Graham Bell Association for the Deaf.

PASCOE, D. P. (1978). An approach to hearing aid selection. *Hearing Instruments, 12* (36).

SHAPIRO, I. (1976). Hearing aid fitting by prescription. *Audiology, 15,* 163-173.

SHORE, I., BILGER, R. D., & HIRSH, I. J. (1960). Hearing aid evaluation: reliability of repeated measures. *J. Speech Hearing Dis., 25,* 152-170.

VICTOREEN, J. A. (1973). Basic principles of otometry. Charles C. Thomas, 163-172.

WALLENFELS, H. B. (1967). Hearing aids on prescription. Springfield: Thomas.

WATSON, N. A., & KNUDSON, V. O. (1940). Selective amplification in hearing aids. *J. Acoust. Soc. Amer., 406-419.*

V

PRINCIPLES OF OTOMETRY

M. DUNCAN MacALLISTER

A compilation of information and procedures assembled and edited by M. Duncan MacAllister, Ph.D., President, Emtech Laboratories, Inc., from various writings of John A. Victoreen, LLD; Lee A. Melen, MS, CCC-A; and Robert W. Hartenstein, MS, CCC-A, with permission.

INTRODUCTION

No chapter on Otometric Procedures would be complete without a reference to that learned gentleman from whose prolific brain "Otometry" had its beginning, the late John A. Victoreen, LLD, Physicist, Inventor, Scientist, Author, Lecturer, Teacher and, among numerous other things, "The Father of Otometry!"

Over the last twenty-five or so years, a majority of the teachings of that great man have been adopted in one way or other, into the battery of procedures and the lexicon of descriptions used in our discipline of hearing prosthetics. Even his detractors, and through the years there were some of those, would have to admit to using, today, many of "Dr. John's" principles.

To those of us who have labored for so many years with the late Dr. Victoreen, in expanding upon, and helping prove those principles, there has been a tendency to climb up, so-to-speak, upon that proverbial soap-box, and shout our findings to all within earshot. Our exuberant enthusiasm not withstanding, to those who have taken up the practice of Otometry, there is left no doubt as to its merits. Therefore, we are pleased to present in the following page, an introduction to Otometric Procedures.

CHAPTER OBJECTIVES

This presentation is intended to describe a field of science which may be called Otometry. In our present discussion this includes only that information which may be needed in deciding the usefulness of a hearing instrument from a strictly acoustical viewpoint. After all, a hearing instrument having no acoustical usefulness would have little other value. Acoustical considerations are presented which are based on the physics of sound pressure transmission and reception as they apply to prosthetics. For present purposes this would refer only to effects which take place at or outside the eardrum with the single exception of loudness sensation. The intention is to show how loudness sensation itself may be used in otometric measurements as a yes or no indicator. It is then being used in exactly the same way that a null indicating meter pointer would be used in other measuring methods. The amount of sensation or deflection is held constant and not considered.

In otometry, and the hearing process in general, everything depends upon the "kind" of sound pressure signal being received. Hearing involves signal processing and analysis in very complex ways all of which occur in the internal side of the eardrum. Variations in instantaneous applied signal pressures contain the intelligibility which is to be extracted. Present hearing instruments are applied to the *external* side of the eardrum. For this reason we should confine our present discussion to those things which are purely acoustical in nature. It is the intention to show that it is possible to make measurements which minimize those effects in the hearing process which are connected with signal processing. This can be done by the choice of a simple technique using a suitable signal presented at discrete signal frequencies.

LIMITATIONS OF OTOMETRY

The integrity of otometry can only be preserved by using signals and methods which can be mathematically described. Some mathematical expressions will be shown here, not because calculations of this kind are needed in the practice of otometry, but to show that it is a science for the most part, and not an art in itself. Without a firm foundation a science cannot attain eventual acceptance in the scientific community or professional community. Sooner or later otometry will have to merge with one of the professions, or become a profession itself.

Like the gold in Ft. Knox gives backing to our monetary system, mathematics gives otometry a firm foundation without having to be constantly used.

Analysis of the word otometry conveys the fact that certain specific things are being done. Otometry may be considered as a tool which may be used by anyone. It can be used to measure and analyze the acoustical effects obtained for an ear through the application of a prosthetic device. It is a means of measuring acoustical ear function without dependence on the kind of hearing impairment or make of hearing instrument involved.

Otometry does not presume to tell anyone *how* to dispense hearing instruments. It merely enables anyone to know *what* an aided ear does. Like a magnifying glass it enables anyone to take a close look at the acoustical part of hearing prosthetics. It is tacitly assumed that all other professional expertise is being followed and applied before otometry is utilized.

Otometry is a science based on numerical standards of comparison which apply only under specified conditions. It should be used to enhance other professional efforts. It is not expected that it should replace them.

BASIC CONSIDERATIONS OF OTOMETRY

Much of otometric practice is based on three considerations:

(1) It has been shown elsewhere that loudness sensation for the non-deficient ear is almost completely independent of signal frequency at some pressure level in the center of the useful pressure range.

(2) There must exist a set of pressures for an ear which would be considered as most comfortable loudness pressures.

(3) That these principles may be applied to objective measurements.

It remains only to define acceptably what is meant by the "center of the pressure range" in order to create a useful standard of comparison between what might be considered as a functionally deficient ear and a non-deficient ear at normally used sound pressure levels.

It would appear to be correct to say that the center of the useful range exists between those signals which are judged by the listener to be "loud" and those which have been judged to be "soft". It would also appear to be logical to assume that these "center-loudness pressures" (CLP) would also be the "most-comfortable-loudness pressures" (MCLP). It would not be proper to ask a listener to locate those pressures which are most comfortable because this would be a subjective opinion of loudness magnitude.

Practical application of these principles shows that there is a small region of uncertainty existing between signals that are judged to be loud or soft without considering *how* loud they are. The region of uncertainty is of the order of several decibels. The center of this region defines the objective center-loudness pressure which corresponds to subjective most-comfortable-loudness pressure. Subjective measurements confirm this.

Validity of the definition of CLP and MCLP may be further verified by making a set of equal-loudness-pressure (ELP) measurements at and between all selected signal frequencies at the CLP "level". It will be found that CLP values are the same as ELP values at the same pressure "level".

Otometry may be found useful for strictly diagnostic purposes for those who may wish to use it to analyze acoustical ear function. It may also be used in the strictly acoustical dispensing of hearing instruments where aided free field measurements are made of prosthetic need without enquiry into the details of the hearing impairment.

BLACK BOX CONCEPT

It is often desirable in scientific work to simplify functional analysis by isolating separate functions and measuring them one at a time. For example, complex systems such as an ear may be treated like a black box having unknown contents with an entrance port and a suitable indicator. One may liken such a box to an ear using a sound pressure input and a loudness sensation output. We can then make perfectly analogous measurements which will clarify ear function for prosthetic analysis. Measurements so made are analogous only when carefully designed to isolate individual properties in a correct way. For example, in the present case the input to the black box would be a single frequency sound pressure signal and the output would be indicated by the listener as a loudness sensation.

What is desired for prosthetics is a knowledge of *where* the center pressures are and *how* the loudness sensation changes with sound pressure at a given signal frequency. A knowledge of acoustics tells us that there are two directions to go because there are two variables and one fixed parameter and that is signal frequency. Only one variable can be changed at a time. We can measure the change in loudness as the sound pressure is varied while signal frequency is held constant or we can hold the sound pressure constant and vary the signal frequency. In either of these cases one would have to measure the sensation of loudness created. We don't want to do this because that would be a subjective opinion we wish to avoid. We can get around this objection by holding the loudness sensation constant and recording the sound pressure change that has to be delivered to produce a constant loudness sensation at each different signal frequency.

It can be seen from the black box principle that we cannot find out what we would like to know about either the box or the ear by using a complex signal. It is essential to use a single frequency signal to isolate the information so that it can be expressed mathematically.

MATHEMATICAL RELATIONS

Measurements made with young adults show that the desired relationships can be expressed in the form of eq. 1 which applies to the whole range of useful pressures and signal frequencies:

$$P_f = P_L \times A_f$$

eq. 1

Where

P_f is defined as the constant (or equal) loudness pressure at frequency, f.

P_L is the sound pressure at a "level", L, (with respect to 1000 Hz.) to which measurements of P_f will be referred. P_f values will vary differently with various signal frequencies at high and low pressure "levels".

The term, A, is shown to vary with frequency, f.

Procedure for calculating the values of the term, A, for various pressure "levels" and signal frequencies is given elsewhere.

There is a pressure level, P_L, at which equation 1, yields values which are almost independent of signal frequency from 11 to 22,000 cycles per second. When measured as an average value representing a small group of supposedly non-deficient teenagers, P_f becomes independent of frequency at about .789 microbars or 72 dB re .0002 microbar. These are the calculated central-loudness pressures.

Subjective evaluations have shown that the 72 dB "level" corresponds to most-comfortable-loudness pressures. These, in turn, correspond to an *objective* estimation of center-loudness pressures.

GRAPHIC ILLUSTRATION OF ACOUSTICAL EAR FUNCTION

Values calculated by means of eq. 1, when plotted appear as shown in figure 1. For a non-deficient ear the center-loudness pressures are conspicuous by their frequency independence. The center-loudness pressures are the only ones which are of *direct* interest prosthetically because this is the pressure region where listening will be concentrated.

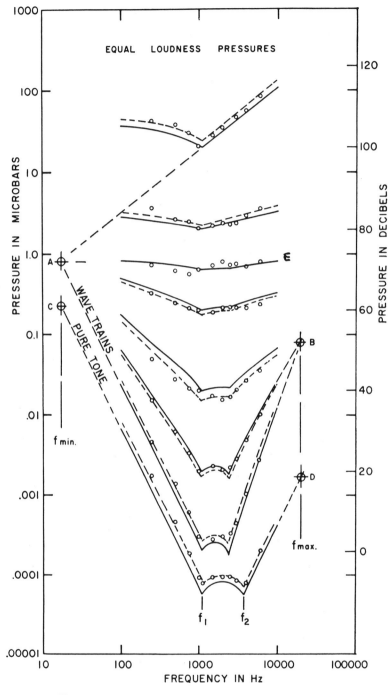

Fig. 1.

The graphs of Figure 1 intersect at the far ends of the frequency range. Pressure and frequency values at the point of intersection are the constants from which the values of the term A, of Figure 1 may be calculated.

So far, we have been discussing a way to describe how ear function may be expressed. What is being presented applies only when decaying wavetrain signals are used. We have shown how a non-deficient ear responds to measurement. We have therefore established a basis upon which we can proceed to relate hearing deficiencies to possible acoustical correction.

For acoustical prothetics a deficient ear may be stated to be one which differs in functionability from a non-deficient ear. In other words a set of graphs measured for a particular deficient ear will differ from those of the young adults shown by Figure 1.

HEARING DEFICIENCY

Ears change with time through environmental exposure. Figure 2 shows a typical individual case, with a change which may occur in 5 to 10 years of exposure to a very noisy environment. At this stage the individual is unaware of a hearing problem. Assuming that we take 1100 Hz. as a point of reference, f, it may be observed that a definite break in graph shape occurs at points corresponding to $1/4f$, $1/2f$, $1f$, and $2f$. Figure 2 differs from the graphs in figure 1, by the difference calculated by eq. 2.

$$P_f = P_L (A \times B)_f + C$$

eq. 2

Changes observed in the response of the ear are found to be explained by a change in the constants comprising the terms, B and C. It is interesting to note that the frequency values 275, 1100, 2200 and 4400 appear to be generally universal and apply to both very small and very large deficiencies of different kinds.

DEFICIENCY CORRECTION

Measured values of CLP for an unaided ear would be compared to similar values for an average unaided non-deficient ear to find the amount of *hearing deficiency* which exists. We are not, however, concerned with the deficiency. We are only concerned with the amount of *sound pressure correction* which will be required to compensate for the deficiency. There is a difference.

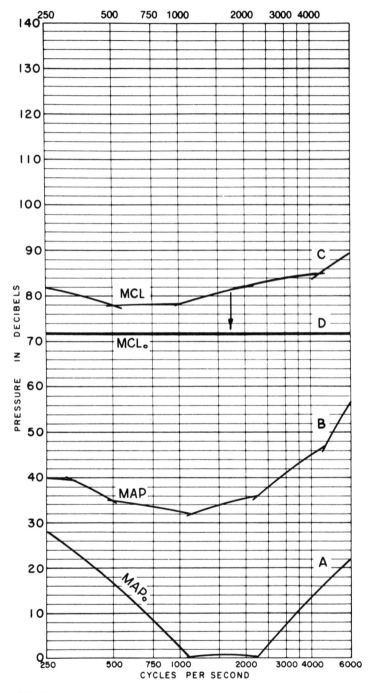

Fig. 2.

Hearing instruments have a large and frequency dependent insertion loss when applied to an ear. The amount of insertion loss varies from ear to ear so that it is not possible to predict in a practical way what it will be. It is apparent that hearing instruments must first supply their own insertion losses. They must do this before they can start to supply the additional pressures needed by the ear to make up for lost loudness sensitivity.

One may eliminate consideration of insertion losses entirely by measuring CLP for a deficient ear with a standardized hearing instrument in place on the ear and operating it at an approximately most-comfortable-loudness "level". This is called a substitution method. By this method, it is merely necessary to refer needed pressures to the calibration of the standardized instrument to see how much more or less than these pressures will be required to meet any pre-determined acoustical objective. It is a rapid and accurate method.

The substitution method has the advantage that aided free-field measurements can be compared directly with unaided free-field measurements of a non-deficient ear. Conclusions drawn from this comparison may be expressed in relation to a few pre-defined axiomatic relationships.

BASIC AXIOMS

(1) The ear is a free-field sound-pressure operated loudness sensation generator.

(2) A hearing instrument is a sound pressure operated sound pressure generator placed between a source of sound pressure signals and the ear canal.

(3) Hearing instruments do not deliver sound pressure signals where they are usually received.

(4) At a given signal frequency, the loudness sensation generated by an ear may be increased by aiding the ear with a hearing instrument which increases received sound pressures.

(5) Prosthetic measurements of a deficient ear must be taken under free-field conditions with a hearing instrument in place in order to properly compare such measurements with those for an unaided non-deficient ear.

(6) Functional usefulness of the ear with respect to acoustical properties will require that the amount of amplification to be applied will be considered separately for each signal frequency.

(7) Signals used must be capable of mathematical description and of providing measurements with mathematical significance.

(8) The standard of comparison for prosthetic purposes should be an average unaided non-deficient ear to which free-field signals are presented in an acceptable manner.

(9) The sound pressure measurements should be made at a pressure "level" where listening would be expected to occur.

LOUDNESS AND SOUND PRESSURES

Loudness is a function of sound pressure applied to the ear at a specified point of delivery. Loudness and sound pressure may be described in terms of each other. For example, the sound pressure of a given signal can be lowered until the signal is no longer of sufficient loudness to be heard. The pressure recorded at this point is called the *threshold pressure*. Threshold pressures are in fact zero loudness pressures. One can also tabulate a series of measured threshold pressures, each taken at a different signal frequency. Such a set of sound pressures may also be called a set of *equal loudness pressures* measured at minimum audible pressures (MAP), where the ear ceases to function. It is better to measure ear function at CLP "level" where the ear will be forced to operate in practice.

Both CLP and MAP measurements meet the requirements of minimum subjective involvement when using a description based on sound pressure signal amplitude and its rate of change.

The actual measured values of loudness pressures obtained for a particular unaided ear will differ with the "kind" of signal being used depending upon how the instantaneous pressure alternations change with time.

The kind of signal which is most desirable for measuring practical acoustic ear function is firmly dictated by demands which have been forced upon the measurement by necessity.

If we are to progress beyond empirical methods and generalities, we must make the assumption that out of all the possibilities there will be but one most desirable set of correction factors for each deficient ear. We must also assume that these should be attained for the user by the dispenser.

It should be safe to use the functional properties of an average young non-deficient ear as an example of what a perfect prosthetic correction might desirably attempt to provide for a deficient ear after being aided.

When making a comparison of this kind, the description should be limited to simple and clear definitions of how ears and hearing instruments function together. As previously described, there are only three numerical terms which can be used to describe and unite ear function and hearing instrument capabilities for purposes of prosthetic comparison. These are:

(1) Loudness sensation generated by the ear,

(2) Sound pressure generated by the instrument, and

(3) Frequency of the signal applied to the ear.

Description of ear function in aided operation should be limited to these three terms. We may, in this way, direct effort to correcting the *causes* of hearing difficulties rather than to try to correct for *effects* which are observed to occur as a result of the deficiency.

SIGNALS

Concealed within the terms "sound pressure" and "alternation rate" is the dimension which gives character to an acoustical signal and describes the "kind" of signal it is. This is *time*. Simple signals differ from each other in "kind" by the time it takes for one single cycle of sound pressure to alternate between maximum and minimum values. Usually this leads to conception and use of continuous pure tone signals of relatively long duration for measuring purposes. Signal duration time, however, loses meaning for signals of very long duration. The ear is not intended to deal with continuous signals or very long signals. Fatigue occurs and it changes with signal length. This alters the sensitivity of the ear to sound pressure signals being received. It is desirable to eliminate such effects when measurements are to be made of practical ear function. This can be done by delivering the optimum number of cycles in the signal.

How long in time should signal duration be? No longer than necessary for recognition. Obviously, signal duration will vary with the number of cycles per second being delivered. About 6 cycles per signal is enough. What this tells us is that for some purposes, we should use signals which all have the same number of cycles per signal not the same time duration per signal as the frequency is changed.

We have stated that for present purposes, a suitable signal should contain a small but constant number of cycles. In this case, the length or duration time of the signal need not be mentioned. It can always be calculated from the signal frequency, or rate of change, if desired. But there is no reason to do this. Had we used a pure tone signal instead, the number of cycles per signal would have varied inversely with signal frequency. This would have lead to an entirely different kind of measurement and to considerably different measured values. Loudness sensation changes with the number of cycles which are presented. The same is true for signals of any constant duration length presented. It applies not only to pure tone signals but also to narrow band noise signals as well as warble tones, etc. Complex signals of any kind, including those of speech, cannot be used for prosthetic measurement purposes because they contain *many* individual frequency components and therefore cannot supply information on a discrete or single frequency basis.

TIME AS A DIMENSION

Time has been shown to be a necessary part of signal description. But used in this way, it merely defines the *rate* per second at which the signal pressure alternates during signal presentation. In connection with rate of change, time is relative. There is no mention of any particular time. Time is simply a way of referring to a kind of signal.

Time is also a necessary part of pressure definition but in a different way. Sound pressure ''levels'' are ''averages'' and they cannot be added together. Sound pressures are constantly varying between maximum positive and negative values. Two or more sound pressures can only be added and specified at some particular instant of time. Instantaneous pressures are the only pressures that can be added together.

OTOMETRIC SIGNALS

Signals suitable for present measuring purposes have a constant and repeatable number of cycles and are called *wavetrain* signals.

In decaying wavetrain signals, the decay rate is not specified. It is the percent of amplitude retained in each succeeding cycle which is specified. A loss of 10% per cycle indicates that 90% is left so that the decrement is then specified as being equal to 0.90.

The decaying (or damped) wavetrain signal used for the acoustical measurements being discussed is shown in Figure 3. This signal decreases to about $1/2$ amplitude in 6 cycles. The spectral distribution is constant throughout the signal presentation, shown in Figure 4.

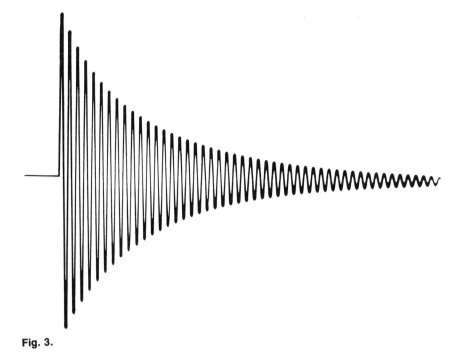

Fig. 3.

PROSTHETIC FITTING TECHNIQUES:

Lee A. Melen, in his paper "Application of Otometric Principles in Binaural Hearing Aid Fittings", has presented a clear picture of all that is necessary in the Otometric technique. This came after several years of practice of otometric fitting and many hundreds of cases at the Guthrie Clinic, in Sayre, Pennsylvania. He describes a hearing instrument, and says, "A sound (sound pressure signal) enters the microphone opening of the hearing instrument, its amplitude is changed, and it is delivered via an appropriate connection to the ear canal. A quality hearing instrument will not change the frequency of the incoming signal, and will not add appreciable distortion to the incoming signal. Its main job is to amplify the sound field (whether it is a body-worn, post-auricular, eyeglass, or in-the-ear instrument). Therefore, any aided measurements must of necessity be made with the instrument in the position it will be worn."

For average sound pressure inputs (65-75 dB re: .0002 dynes/cm^2), the normal ear operates "flat" across the frequency range. It has been

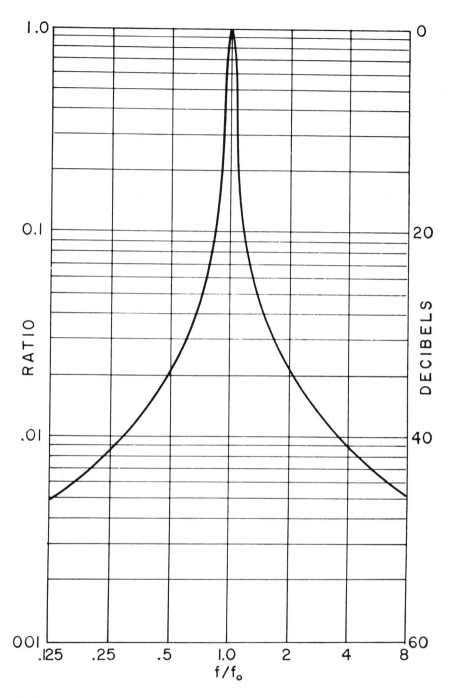

Fig. 4.

experimentally shown that for inputs of 72 dB, using a damped wave-train signal having a decrement of 0.90, most comfortable loudness is created in the normal ear (Figure 5). Thus, we see equal loudness at equal sound pressures for all frequencies across the range measured (250-6000 Hz). This has also been shown to be a curve describing the locus of central loudness pressure. A normal hearing individual prefers to listen to sound when it is not too loud, and not too soft.

The relationship between threshold (minimum audible) sound pressures and central loudness pressures in a hearing-impaired ear is drastically changed from the relationship of the two in a normal ear. The change is unpredictable, and therefore, pressures which evoke central loudness in an impaired ear cannot be predicted from threshold measurements in the impaired ear. Most comfortable loudness pressures must be measured directly in every ear, as the central loudness pressure locus.

Since we do not usually listen to sounds at the threshold of audibility, but indeed, do most of our listening at levels in the average sound pressure range of 65-75 dB (for speech and many other sounds as well), the prosthetic correction of hearing impairment must attempt to re-establish normal relationships between frequency, sound pressure, and loudness in this range. Therefore, the first PROSTHETIC OBJEC-TIVE becomes immediately clear: The aided hearing-impaired ear must respond to inputs of approximately 72 dB, using a suitable discreet frequency signal, at a most desirable loudness. If a deficient ear can be made to do this, it will be shown to behave exactly as a normal ear in this sound pressure range, at which most listening is done.

Instrumentation for these measurements is commercially available. A free-field sound pressure generator, called an Equaton Sound Pressure Comparator, and a Otomet Free Field Generator, creates discreet-frequency (.25, .5, .75, 1, 2, 2.5, 3, 4, and 6 KHz) signals having the waveform shown in figure 3.

The waveform is called a damped wavetrain. If differs from a conventional pure-tone in that each succeeding cycle of the wavetrain is damped, or decreases by a given factor, in amplitude. Thus, the relative spectral distribution of the energy in the signal will be the same at the nth cycle regardless of frequency. The few cycles presented per signal prevent auditory fatigue and adaptation, which has been shown to be frequency-dependent, and which occurs with the use of pure tones. In addition, the signal may be employed in an ordinary room, in that its short duration prevents the creation of standing waves and unpredictable amounts of sound pressure at different points of the sound field.

The method employed is a simple scientific substitution method. A personal earmold is made for the ear to be measured, and is coupled to a

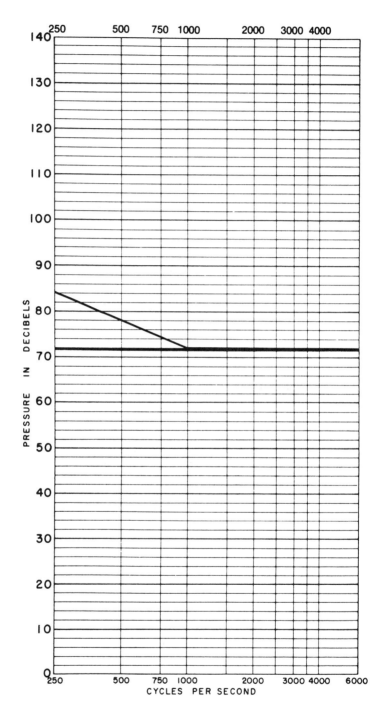

Fig. 5.

laboratory standard hearing instrument in the normal fashion. The laboratory standard instrument is a normal hearing aid whose parameters are exactly known by measurement in a hearing instrument analyzer. It is an instrument whose parameters can be modified as necessary by the manufacturer to fulfill the prescriptive measurements.

The ear to be measured is fitted with a custom-made earmold, and suitably connected to the hearing instrument. The individual is seated at 28″ on axis with the free-field speaker which will present the signals. The hearing instrument is turned on and is referenced to a 72 dB input at 1000 Hz (the middle of the frequency range). This is simply done by variably presenting signals of more or less than 72 dB and asking the individual to say "loud" or "soft." Some adjustment of the volume control of the hearing instrument is necessary at this point to ensure that for a 72 dB 1000 Hz signal, loudness where loud and soft converge (MCLP) has been attained. Most individuals have been seen to have a "comfortable" loudness range of about ±4 dB, with most comfortable loudness located in the central part of the range.

With the volume control of the hearing instrument now set in the reference position, signals of other frequencies are presented in the same manner. The "comfortable" loudness range, or central part of the range, is plotted on the otometric chart. Maximum tolerable pressures are found by presenting increasingly higher sound pressure signals at each frequency to the limits of the equipment (100 dB free-field) or until a threshold of discomfort is reached. If a threshold of discomfort is reached before the limits of the equipment, the input sound pressure plus the gain of the instrument may be used to specify the maximum tolerable pressure at that frequency.

As mentioned earlier, the first prosthetic objective is to create aided most comfortable loudness listening pressure values of 72 dB for each frequency. Because of the effects of upward spread of masking, relative predominance of low frequency sounds in the environment, and relative lesser importance of low frequency sounds for speech intelligibility, the low frequency aided comfortable loudness values are "rolled-off" at a rate of 3 dB/octave for each 10 dB of in-use gain at 1000 Hz. Hence the overall prosthetic objective will look like the graph in Figure 5.

Each ear is measured for its amplification needs in the same fashion, with the opposite ear suitably occluded if necessary. In this fashion, bilateral prosthetic correction will provide equal central loudness pressure values for a given input of sound pressure signal from the midline, and hence maintain or restore the possibility of stereophonic perception of sound (provided the more central binaural functions are intact).

The laboratory test instrument is then taken from the measured ear, with volume control at the reference position, and measured into a 2 cc coupler in a hearing instrument analyzer. The amount of in-use gain is then determined in the usual fashion, subtracting input from output at each frequency.

Any deviation from the prosthetic objective in measured central loudness pressure values is then appropriately added or subtracted from the 2 cc coupler frequency response of the instrument, and the prescription is written. Measured maximum tolerable pressures (maximum power output of the hearing instrument) are specified if necessary, with the amount of in-use gain at 1000 Hz. The prescription can be filled by forwarding it to the manufacturer, who selects an instrument with the prescribed response from stock, or in the absence of an already manufactured instrument satisfying the requirements, manufactures one to the specified response. The prescribed instrument will be the same model as the laboratory standard instrument, in order to eliminate all possible sources of error due to microphone type and placement, circuitry differences, etc.

The prescription can usually be met by the manufacturer, with the exception of two limitations: 1) an ear which demonstrates a "breakpoint," after which no useful pitch discrimination exists (frequency information will probably not be decoded), and 2) a frequency response which is an electronic impossibility. These two limitations have been seen on occasion, but extremely rarely. It then becomes a question of accepting a prosthetic compromise, i.e., to do what is prosthetically possible and use a hearing instrument despite the fact that it cannot meet the prosthetic objective entirely.

An example of otometric prescriptive procedures, with otometric charts, for a real ear, is shown in Figures 5 through 11.

Average measurement time with a co-operative adult patient is approximately 30 minutes for binaural measurements, each ear measured separately. If difficulties are encountered, it may be desirable to further study the loudness functions of an ear in greater detail, both unaided and aided, in the free field and under earphones.

Measurement to remeasurement variability has been seen to be limited to ± 4 dB for all ears measured (with the exception of fluctuating hearing problems), and ± 2 dB for most ears. Individuals with sensorineural (inner ear) hearing impairments have virtually no difficulty detecting even the smallest changes of sound pressure (2 dB increments), while conductively impaired (outer and middle ear) patients have considerably wider comfortable loudness ranges (± 6-8 dB around central or most comfortable loudness pressures).

Some clinical verification studies have appeared in the literature concerning these points. In addition, further experimental and descriptive works appear in the literature, for the interested reader.

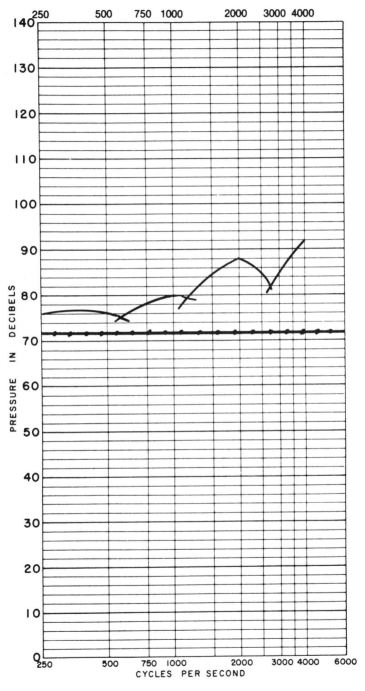

Fig. 6.

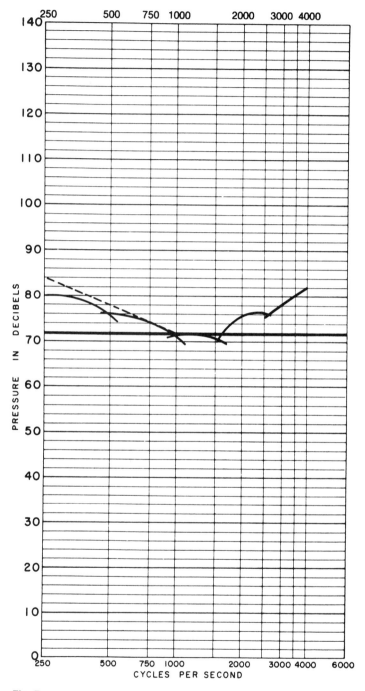

Fig. 7.

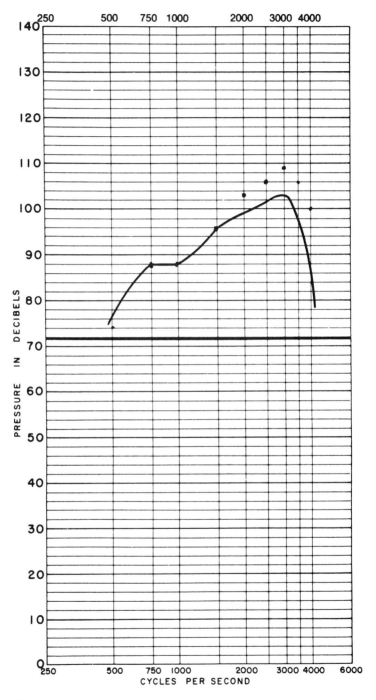

Fig. 8.

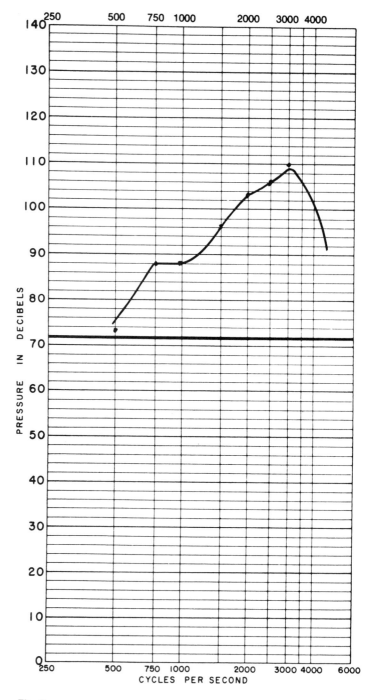

Fig. 9.

PRESCRIPTION TABULATION (DIRECT SUBSTITUTION METHOD)

Frequency	250	500	750	1k	2k	2.5k	3k	4k	6k
Aided MCLP measured values	80	76	74	72	72	76	76	78	
MCLP Objectives	84	78	74	72	72	72	72	72	
Difference	-4	-2	0	0	0	+4	+4	+6	
Test Inst. RDP values (2cc) + diff. = prescription (Rx)	-25	-11	0	0	+8	+11	+14	+15	

Gain at 1000Hz: ___18 dB___

MPO, if different than test Inst._____

    Ear: Right____   Left _X___

    Hearing Inst. type: Post-Auricular _X_   Body_____

             Eyeglass_____   In-The-Ear_____   Canal_____

    Manufacturer:_____

    Model_____

    Receiver:_____

    Connector type_____

    Telephone switch_ _No___

Fig. 10. Prescription tabulation for patient S.M. Left Ear.

Figure 11 Courtesy of J. Michael Canary, Annapolis, Md.

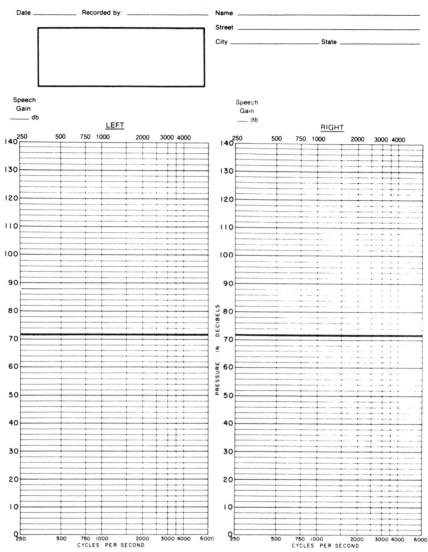

Fig. 11.

OTOMETRIC PROCEDURES

Otometric Objective - To correct the loudness deficiency in deficient ears to the Central Loudness Pressure (CLP) at which the components of speech are most comfortably heard at each discreet signal frequency in both ears so that stereophonic perception is achieved.

PATIENT: _____

DATE: _____ AGE: _____

Recommended unaided measurements prior to Direct Substitution
(To be made on separate sound pressure charts for each ear, if desired)

1.) Unaided free-field CLP each ear separately, with other ear occluded.
2.) MAP (each ear)
3.) Unaided MTP. (each ear)
4.) Frequency discrimination. (each ear)

Manufacturer, _____

Model, & Serial # _____

Frequency setting _____

Gain _____ Output _____

Mold type _____

Filter type _____

Receiver & Connector _____

DIRECT SUBSTITUTION

1.) **AIDED CLP** (free field) with temporary test instrument and final custom mold. Adjust sound pressure to 72dB reference at 1000 Hz each ear separately with other occluded. (Do not move gain control after reference is obtained.)

COMMENTS: _____

_____

_____

2.) **DIFFERENCE** (+ or -) From normal CLP (72dB) - at each signal frequency with temporary test instrument in use.

3.) **IN USE GAIN (ANALYZER)** of test instrument (with aided reference at 72dB at 1000 Hz) - (RDP values - 2cc Coupler).

4.) **TEST INSTRUMENT** "in use gain" (step #3) + difference (step #2) = **PRESCRIPTION** (Rx)

FINAL CONSIDERATIONS

1.) Surplus gain. 2.) Sterophonic perception - CLP both ears aided. 3.) Tolerance - Aided each ear separate. 4.) Low frequency roll off, if any.

COMMENTS: _____

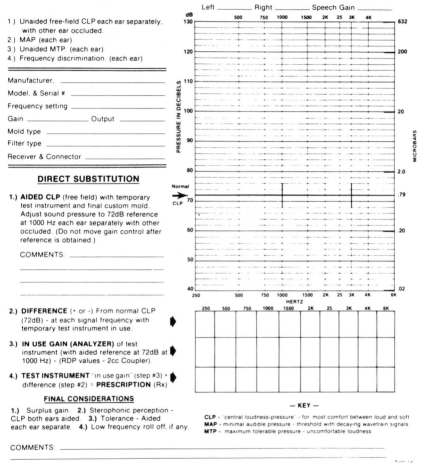

Left _____ Right _____ Speech Gain _____

— KEY —

CLP - "central loudness-pressure" - for most comfort between loud and soft
MAP - minimal audible pressure - threshold with decaying wavetrain signals
MTP - maximum tolerable pressure - uncomfortable loudness

Fig. 12.

To summarize, otometric prescriptive measurements:

1 provide a prosthetic objective which makes the selection and fitting of a hearing instrument relatively simple,

2 are repeatable with surprising accuracy from test to retest,

3 enable the clinician or hearing instrument dispenser to make adjustments on hearing instruments of dissatisfied hearing aid wearers which will then fulfill the prosthetic objective, and

4 can be performed in an ordinary room without the necessity of having a soundproof environment.

VERIFICATION MEASUREMENTS

When measurements with a calibrated laboratory standard hearing instrument have been made, and when the appropriate instrument for each ear has been supplied by the manufacturer, it is possible not only to verify that each instrument functions on the ear as desired, but also that the two instruments operate together in an optimal fashion.

Signals originating from the midline should be perceived by the listener as coming from the center, or straight ahead. With each instrument referenced to MCLP for a 72 dB 1000 Hz signal by the listener, signals are presented at 66 dB from 1000 Hz to 4000 Hz. The listener is asked to close his eyes, and to point to the direction from which the sound apparently originates. If the listener consistently points in one direction, it is known that one of the two instruments is turned on higher than the other. The instruments are referenced again such that equal loudness in both ears has been obtained, and the measurement is repeated. Ideally, all signals should be perceived as originating from the center. If necessary, to achieve this condition, inserts or modification of earmold canal bore, tubing size, and so forth can be used.

When this condition has been achieved, it will be readily seen that any other kind of test for sound source localization can be easily performed by the listener.

A similar measurement can be obtained at or near threshold, or at any other "level" of loudness or signal input in the hearing range.

Binaural summation of loudness can also be accurately assessed, by making both monaural and binaural measurements at various "levels" of loudness and signal input in the hearing range. It has been seen that there is a 6 dB improvement of loudness function around MCLP in the binaural condition as opposed to the monaural condition, and between a 2-4 dB improvement at or around threshold of audibility.

Other tests of "performance" can be made, such as signal detection in controlled ambient noise, speech perception tasks in noise, and so forth, but these cannot be considered "otometric" and should therefore be performed in proper accordance with learning theory.

BINAURAL CANDIDACY:

The question of binaural candidacy has troubled generations of audiologists, hearing aid specialists, ENT physicians, and the consumer public. The question of the integrity of binaural functions is indeed a diagnostic one, and should therefore be dealt with during the diagnostic work-up.

It is probably unwise to preclude the use of binaural amplification even for those individuals who show binaural function deficits during the diagnostic work-up until a fair trial with equal binaural inputs from sound field sources has been obtained. Predictively, however, it might be suspected that these individuals will not fare as well as those with normal binaural function during diagnostic testing. The question cannot be answered in advance, since learning, in the neuro-physiologic sense of the term, is an important factor.

All other individuals with two functional ears and intact binaural functions have simply not received complete prosthetic attention until each ear is measured and provided with a prosthetic device which best re-establishes normal relationships of sound pressure, frequency, and loudness.

A SUMMARY:

A summary of the procedures of Otometric measurement in a "short recipe" form might best be taken from Robert Hartenstein's paper "Clinical Use of Otometry in Hearing Aid Dispensing," by permission:

PROCEDURE:

"Clinical application of Otometric principles provides us with a tool for measuring how an ear or the combination of an ear and a hearing instrument respond. The basic instrumentation for these measurements is a suitable free-field sound pressure generator, producing a damped wave train signal of a decrement of .90 at discrete frequencies from .25-6KHz. At the beginning of the procedure, the patient is seated 28 inches away from the speaker which is placed directly in front, at ear level. The basic format of the evaluation procedure requires the determination of:

1 Unaided free-field 'central loudness pressure' locus, (CLP) each ear separately, with other ear occluded (with ear-plug).

2 Aided free-field 'CLP' locus, each ear separately, with other occluded.

3 Tolerance, each ear separately aided, with opposite occluded.

4 Both ears aided 'CLP' locus, to show if stereophonic perception has been achieved.

The method used is to ask the patient to point to a card which has three words printed on it: 'LOUD,' 'SOFT,' and 'NOTHING.' For children, a large and a small circle on a card may be used. The sound pressure is simply varied in an ascending, descending or a bracketing technique until the patient points to, 'Loud' and 'Soft.' Logically this may be thought of as the 'Most comfortable loudness pressure.' This point is *NOT*, however, subjectively defined by the listener.

The data are plotted on Otometric charts which are in terms of decibels of peak sound pressure 0-140 (re: .0002 dynes/cm^2) and frequency in Hertz (250-6000). Fig. 1, 2, 5, 6, 7, 8, 9. When testing in the aided condition, the gain control (volume control) of the hearing instrument is referenced for 72 dB using a Damped Wave Train at 1000 Hz. Once the gain control is so referenced, it is left untouched at that setting, and signals of other frequencies are then presented and plotted. Clinically we have seen that most people have a range of about ±4 dB between 'Loud' and 'Soft.' From our testing we have demonstrated that the manner of presentation is irrelevant.

Once all measurements have been taken, a prescription may be tabulated by a direct substitution method. This is obtained by taking aided measured values on a *known* or 'standard' hearing instrument and finding the difference between those and the prosthetic objective. Then, the differences are appropriately added to the frequency response to formulate a final prescription. The only arbitrary variation which is incorporated clinically is a low frequency 'roll-off' at a rate of 3 dB/octave for each 10 dB of 'in use gain' at 1000 Hz. Reducing low frequency gain is a way of preventing these signals from over-loading the hearing instrument and simultaneously preventing the effects of upward spreading of a masking effect. At this point, the final prescription is written and forwarded with the order for the instrument to the manufacturer. Once the hearing instrument is obtained, the patient is fitted and otometrically rechecked to make sure the prescription instrument meets the ordered specifications."

Mr. Hartenstein goes on to say,

"A high maximum deliverable pressure should also be incorporated into the hearing instrument when possible. The instantaneous *peak* sound pressures of conversational speech are between 88-92 dB. For example working with an instrument having a gain of 30 dB and having peak inputs of approximately 90 dB, a pressure of 120 dB is achieved. Thus, the instruments we have been using have a maximum deliverable pressure of from 125-132 dB.

Interestingly, we have very few tolerance problems using the maximum deliverable pressure in this area (125-132 dB) when maximum deliverable pressure extends well into the high frequency region. This is due in part to the dB per octave rise which is being incorporated in the hearing instruments, and in part to the proportion of energy appropriated in the lower frequencies compared to that in the higher frequencies."

In concluding this chapter on Otometric Procedures, I'd like to add that it has been shown that the ear, as well as a hearing instrument, operates on a peak to peak basis rather than the Root-Mean-Square (RMS) which we're all so used to using in defining most signals. Mathematically, this represents quite a difference in that peak to peak equals RMS times 2.828, and peak equals RMS times 1.414. Therefore, one can almost always add approximately 20 dB on to audiometric readings of discomfort taken with standard pure-tone and speech signals through most audiometers.

Our concluding subject will address certain ''differences'' in the fitting of All-in-the-ear aids versus the other styles where the ''plumbing'' may be fine tuned for acoustic effects.

The author along with several other of those dispensers who utilize the practice of otometry as the procedure of choice, have found that with the advent of the so-called ''universal'' or ''fit-all'' canal hearing aid and other stock type ITE instruments, it is now possible to utilize the substitution method of Otometry for fitting these types of instruments. The important thing in their use, is the placement in your Electro-acoustic test chamber must approximate that of the manufacturer. In other words, does the manufacturer have the microphone facing into the sound source in his test chamber, or is it at right angles to the source? Does he test with the receiver tubing left extended for a probe, or does he couple to the coupler with a clay-like dough to seal the canal into his coupler? The coupling of an ITE in the acoustic test chamber is a critical point, and can effect the actual frequency response reading by as much as 20 dB. This is especially true in the high frequency areas.

When using a ''universal'' or stock instrument as a standard, it is equally important to note the canal length and order the approximate same length for the final instrument. We have also found that if an ITE or canal aid is ordered with a low frequency pot where possible, the final ''fine tuning'' process is much simpler. Another area of intense interest these days, and one the author has been deeply involved in while doing research for a patent, is that of phase shift and phase relationship using real time analysis and Fast Fourier Transform (FFT), especially in relation to complex signals. All this adds up to a cleaner, more pure amplification without having to add the multitude of parts that are so difficult to ''jam'' into that tiny space in the shell. Otometrically, this measures out as less gain and output needed to do the same job. The future indeed looks fabulous.

In closing, we might add that a new damped wavetrain generator is on the drawing board, with totally electronic attenuators and compatible with computer systems which should be the ultimate equipment for practitioners of Otometric Principles. We have included a reference section for those who wish to study in depth those Otometric Principles and experiences of well-known professionals in Otometric Dispensing.

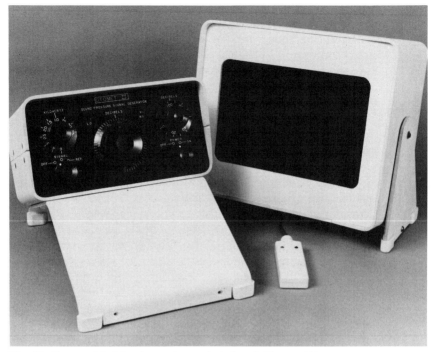

Fig. 13. New model of the damped wave train free field generator.

GLOSSARY

CLP Central Loudness Pressures

MCLP Most Comfortable Loudness Pressures

ELP Equal Loudness Pressures

MAP Minimum Audible Pressure

MTP Maximum Tolerable Pressure

MDP Maximum Deliverable Pressure

MDO Maximum Deliverable Output

MPO Maximum Pressure Output

RDP Relative Delivered Pressures

DWT Damped Wave-Train

Roll-off An added attenuation of amplitude in the low frequency range (100 Hz through 750 Hz, up to but not including 1000 Hz).

FFT Fast Fourier Transform, A mathematical series of calculations using calculus and now-a-days, through the miracle of computers built into real-time analyzers, accomplished in literal seconds, compared to the hours and even days necessary on slide rules just a decade or two ago.

RMS Root Mean Square—The average value obtained by taking the square root of the arithmetic mean of the squares of the set values, given by:

$$V_{RMS} = \sqrt{\frac{V_1^2 + V_2^2 \ldots\ldots V_N^2}{n}}$$

where v_1, v_2, ... v_n are the values to be averaged, n is the number of values, and v_{rms} the root-mean-square value.

REFERENCES

BRUCE, PETER. Measurement of Most Comfortable Loudness Pressures with a Non-verbal Population Through the use of Damped Wave-Train Signals, January, 1978.

CROUCH, J. D., and PENDRY, B. L. Otometry in Clinical Hearing Aid Dispensing, *Hearing Aid Journal*, Sept., 1975, and Oct., 1975.

GAENSLEN, GEORGE R. A Report on Otometry, *Hearing Aid Journal*, March, 1973.

————— . Fitting a Hearing Aid is an Exact Science, *Hearing Aid Journal*, August, 1975.

HARTENSTEIN, ROBERT W. Clinical Use Of Otometry In Hearing Aid Dispensing. The Hammond Clinic, May, 1978.

MACALLISTER, M. DUNCAN. Professional Dispensing through Otometry. Vicon Inst. Company, 1979.

MELEN, LEE A. Prescriptive Prosthetic Applications of Otometric Sound Pressure Measurements in the Selection and Fitting of Hearing Instruments. *Annals of Otology, Rhinology & Laryngology*, 1977.

————— . Application of Otometric Principles in Binaural Hearing Aid Fittings. Project 76-12 Guthrie Foundation for Medical Research, 1976.

MELEN, LEE A. HFHG Earmold, *Hearing Aid Journal*, March, 1978.

MELEN, LEE A. Otometry, An Emerging Prosthetic Discipline, *Guthrie Bulletin*, Vol. 47, Summer, 1977.

————— . Selection and Fitting of Hearing Instruments—A Prosthetic, Not Diagnostic Task, *Audecibel*, Spring, 1978.

PRATT, LINDSAY; MELEN, LEE A., and MOORE, R. Studies in Otometric Fitting of Hearing Instruments, 1978.

VICTOREEN, JOHN A. Lecture Note Series, Victoreen Laboratory, 1973.

————. Equal Loudness Pressures Determined with a Decaying Oscillatory Waveform, *JASA*, Vol. 55, 2, Feb., 1974.

VICTOREEN, JOHN A. Basic Principles of Otometry, CC Thomas, 1973.

————. Hearing Enhancement, CC Thomas, 1960.

————. Hearing Instruments and Loudness, *Audecibel*, Fall, 1972.

————. The Prescription of Hearing Instruments, *Audecibel*, Spring, 1968.

————. Basic Otometric Principles, *Audecibel*, Spring, 1963.

————. The Practice of Otometry, paper delivered at International Hearing Aid Seminar, San Diego, 1975.

————. Hearing Instrument Dispensing by Prescription, paper delivered at New Mexico ENT Society Meeting, Sept., 1975.

————. Otometry at Its Purpose, Otomet Corporation, 1977.

————. Principles of Hearing Prosthetics, Otomet Corporation, 1977.

————. Elements of Otometry, Otomet Corporation, 1977.

————. A Technical Basis for Professional Hearing Instrument Dispensing, 1978.

————. Measurement of Acoustical Ear Function, 1978.

————. A Mathematical Basis for Hearing Prosthetics, Otomet Corporation, 1978.

VICTOREEN, ROBERT R. The Otometric Hearing Instrument, *Hearing Aid Journal*, March, 1968.

VI

APPLICATION OF PROBE MICROPHONES FOR VALIDATING HEARING AID FITTINGS

DAVID A. PREVES

INTRODUCTION

The issue of how to best validate a hearing aid fitting has been a problem dating back to the early days of hearing aids. The methodology of hearing aid fitting validation has become inextricably intertwined with the method of choosing the electroacoustic performance of a hearing aid for a particular hearing impaired individual. Thus, the particular validation method employed depends heavily on what criteria constitute a successful fitting for the particular hearing aid selection method utilized.

Hearing aid selection methods generally fall into the comparative category, or the traditional hearing aid evaluation procedure, and the prescriptive category, which uses a formula to select hearing aid performance from audiological and patient history data. The comparative hearing aid evaluation technique involves selecting the "best" hearing aid for a patient by comparing speech discrimination scores for different hearing aids worn by that patient. The comparative method has been widely criticized for being unreliable and insensitive for the differentiation of hearing aids (Shore et al., 1960; Thorton and Raffin, 1978; Studebaker, 1982; Schwartz, 1982). It has been found that performance scoring with different hearing aids using auditory speech discrimination tests does not necessarily correspond to differences in amplification between hearing aids primarily because the number of test items is too small. The result is that test-retest repeatability differences in discrimination scores are often greater than those differences in discrimination scores caused by the hearing aids themselves. To make these speech discrimination tests more reliable, many more test items would have to be utilized, which would result in excessively long testing time. The problems associated with the comparative approach of hearing aid selection led to the development of prescriptive hearing aid fitting approaches.

Although the prescriptive approach for hearing aid selection dates back several decades (Lybarger, 1944; Watsen and Knudsen, 1940), this type of methodology did not receive widespread serious consideration until the 1960's and early 1970's (Lybarger, 1963; Millin, 1965; Reddell and Calvert, 1966; Markle and Zaner, 1966; Wallenfels, 1967; Seiler, 1971; Martin, 1973; Brooks, 1973; Victoreen, 1973; Pascoe, 1975). Continuing the trend, several prescriptive methods for recommending the electroacoustic performance of hearing aids have been advocated within the last decade (Berger, 1976; Shapiro, 1976; Byrne and Tonnison, 1976; Pascoe, 1978; Skinner et al., 1982; Mason and Popelka, 1982; McCandless and Lyregaard, 1983; DeJonge, 1985; Libby, 1985; Cox, 1985; Byrne and Dillon, 1986).

This recent proliferation of prescriptive hearing aid fitting approaches has made it necessary to find viable methods to validate whether hearing aids are fulfilling prescriptions on an individual basis. Several of these prescriptive fitting methods estimate from audiological and patient history data the real ear gain which a hearing instrument should provide in situ (Berger, 1976; Pascoe, 1978; McCandless and Lyregaard, 1983; DeJonge, 1985; Mason and Popelka, 1982; Cox, 1985; Byrne and Dillon, 1986). Many of these prescriptive hearing aid fitting methods utilize a real ear measurement called functional gain for validation. Functional gain is an assessment of how much a hearing aid improves a hearing aid wearer's hearing threshold levels relative to the unaided condition. Functional gain is simply the difference between the unaided hearing threshold levels and the aided hearing threshold levels. Many of the prescription methods referred to above predict the aided hearing thresholds that should be produced by an effective hearing aid fitting on a particular patient.

Although the validation of real ear gain provided by a hearing aid in accordance to these prescription methods has been traditionally accomplished by measuring the functional gain, recently, the electroacoustic measurement of insertion gain with a probe microphone system has been utilized as an estimate of functional gain. Insertion gain is a measure of how much a hearing aid changes the sound pressure level in the hearing aid wearer's ear canal. Thus, insertion gain may theoretically be used also to validate those particular prescription fitting formulae which predict real ear gain.

CHAPTER OBJECTIVES

Several probe-tube microphone systems which perform the insertion gain measurement have been recently introduced. Due to the similarity in features and number of these instruments, selection of a probe microphone system may be a difficult decision-making process. The main purposes of this chapter are:

— to point out what advantages the real ear measurement of insertion gain have over the traditional electroacoustic measures of hearing aid performance

— to examine how a probe microphone system may be used to confirm prescriptive hearing aid fittings

— to clarify terminology associated with *in situ* measurements utilizing probe microphones

— to suggest what features may be desirable in a probe microphone system

— to deliniate several of the various methods of sound field equalization used by probe microphone systems and how they relate to the ANSI and IEC documents from which they have evolved

— to point out some of the pitfalls which may be encountered in making real ear measurements with a probe microphone system

HOW INSERTION GAIN AND FUNCTIONAL GAIN ARE RELATED

The concept of insertion gain was first proposed by Ayers (1953) and further elaborated on by Dalsgaard and Jensen (1976). Insertion gain is the amount by which a hearing aid changes the *sound pressure level* at a point in the external auditory meatus, relative to the unaided condition (Figure 1).

Although the validation of real ear gain provided by hearing aid fittings in accordance with prescription methods has been traditionally accomplished by comparing unaided and aided hearing thresholds to determine the functional gain, there are a few prescriptive methods such as POGO (Prescription of gain/output) (McCandless and Lyregaard, 1983) which utilize insertion gain directly for validation. This is not to say that insertion gain cannot be used to verify those prescription methods which estimate the functional gain or predict aided thresholds. On the contrary, because of the widespread belief that insertion gain and functional gain are equal at least on the average, probe-determined real ear gain is being used increasingly to estimate functional gain, and hence, to verify many prescription fittings.

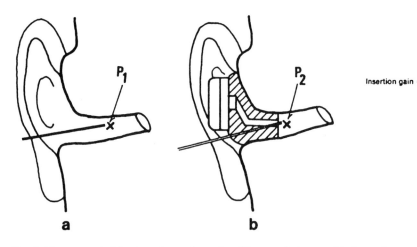

Fig. 1. The concept of the insertion gain as the difference between aided sound pressure P2 (b) and unaided sound pressure P1 (a) in an ear canal (Reprinted with permission) (From Dalsgaard and Jensen, 1976)

One reason for an insertion gain measurement is to estimate the real ear gain provided by a hearing aid without going through the comparatively long process of determining hearing thresholds at audiometric test frequencies. Therefore, an important criterion for the insertion gain measurement is the assumption that it provides an accurate estimate of the functional gain provided by a hearing aid.

There have been many studies examining the question of whether insertion gain is equal to functional gain. Early studies showed that they were about equal, on the average, with a tendency for insertion gain to be greater than functional gain at some frequencies. Also, there could be large differences between the two measures for individuals (Rumoshosky and Preves, 1976; Preves and Orton, 1978). Later studies have confirmed the pattern for *mean equality with large individual variability* between insertion gain and functional gain (Harford, 1984; Arlinger and Jerlvall, 1984; Olsson, 1985; Tecca and Woodford, 1985; Zemplenyi et al.; Dillon and Murray, 1987). For example, the study by Tecca and Woodford showed differences up to 18 dB at 3kHz between insertion gain and functional gain for certain individuals, although the mean difference between the two measures for all 34 subjects was only 0.15 dB.

Killion (1986) has calculated that the agreement between insertion gain and functional gain should produce a standard deviation of 5-7 dB if there is careful control of the many measurement variables that can lead to artifacts. Among the problems encountered in comparing insertion gain to functional gain are:

— Masking from the internal circuit noise of the hearing aid

— environmental noise in the sound room

— subject head movement between aided and unaided conditions

— variation in earmold seating between insertion gain and functional gain measurements

— use of 5 dB attenuator steps for the functional gain measurements

The large standard deviation predicted by Killion of 5-7 dB is in agreement with that found in the studies cited above: assuming a Gaussian (bell-shaped symmetrical) distribution of the data points, a 5 dB standard deviation could be expected to produce up to a 15 dB difference (3 standard deviations) between insertion gain and functional gain for a small but significant percentage of individual hearing aid wearers.

Obviously, the relationship between insertion gain and functional gain does not hold for cases of severe or profound hearing losses in which the hearing thresholds at some frequencies are beyond the range of sound field audiometers. In such cases, an insertion gain measurement at a particular frequency can be determined, but a functional gain may not be measurable.

TRADITIONAL ELECTROACOUSTIC HEARING AID MEASURES

One may think of a hierarchy in terms of levels of realism in the methods available for evaluating the electroacoustic performance of hearing aid fittings (Preves, 1984). This hierarchy ranges from the least realistic 2cc coupler measures to the most realistic in situ real ear measures. Some of the traditional electroacoustic measures of hearing aid performance are less well suited than the *in situ* insertion gain measurement for validating prescriptive fittings. Among these are 2cc coupler measurements, which were originally intended only for quality control purposes at the manufacturing level. The HA-2cc coupler uses an earmold simulator which eliminates from the measurements variations due to differences in earmolds. Variations due to differences in some but not all earmold parameters can be measured with the HA-1 2cc coupler which uses the individual earmold associated with the hearing aid fitting. The HA-1 2cc coupler has been widely used for testing in-the-ear hearing aids. It is not possible to realistically demonstrate the effects of earmold venting variations with the HA-1 2cc coupler due to an artificial resonance formed by the earmold vent and hard-walled coupler volume (Preves, 1977).

A higher level of realism is obtained if an ear simulator such as the modified Zwislocki or IEC711 coupler is substituted for the 2cc coupler. With this type of device, the mean impedance of normal middle ears is presented as the acoustic load for the hearing aid output.

The ear simulator can thus realistically demonstrate the effects of variations in earmold parameters that might occur when worn on median ears. Placing an ear simulator on a manikin such as KEMAR® instead of a hearing aid test chamber produces the next higher level of realism — that of including the effects on hearing aid performance of diffraction caused by the pinna, head and torso of a median person.

Using Correction Factors to Predict Insertion Gain from 2cc Coupler Data

If a stock postauricular hearing aid is used for a fitting, depending on the earmold utilized, it is sometimes possible to get an idea of the insertion gain it will produce on the KEMAR® manikin from the manufacturer's specification sheet. However, individual differences of the wearer's physiology from the KEMAR® manikin and parameters of the particular earmold employed can produce large variations from the insertion gain shown on the specification sheet. With a custom hearing aid, it may be possible to get an idea of the insertion gain it will provide from the use of correction factors to convert the 2cc coupler gain to insertion gain on the KEMAR® manikin (Lybarger and Teder, 1986). As a practical example of the importance of insertion gain, the Veterans Administration requires that all custom in-the-ear hearing aids supplied to VA clinics be accompanied by an estimate or measurement of insertion gain. Manufacturers of custom in-the-ear hearing aids are routinely accomplishing this estimate of insertion gain using a computer-generated frequency response based on tables similar to those given in the Lybarger and Teder article. These estimates are only a first approximation of the real ear insertion gain since they are intended for unvented in-the-ear aids fitted on the KEMAR® manikin. Since the majority of in-the-ear fittings have some type of venting, the correction factor approach may not provide a very close estimate of the actual insertion gain achieved either on the KEMAR® manikin, or on the individual. Figure 2 shows an example of the differences between the estimated insertion gain for an in-the-ear hearing aid from 2cc coupler frequency response taken with the vent closed and the insertion gain of the same hearing aid on the KEMAR® manikin with the vent open. In the final analysis, the real ear measurement of insertion gain with a probe microphone on the individual for whom the hearing aid fitting has been designed should provide the most realistic assessment of electroacoustic performance.

Changes caused by individual anatomical and physiological variations cannot be ascertained with either the KEMAR® manikin or the median correction factors. For example, a standard deviation of up to 5 dB in the higher frequencies was found from the median ear canal SPL produced

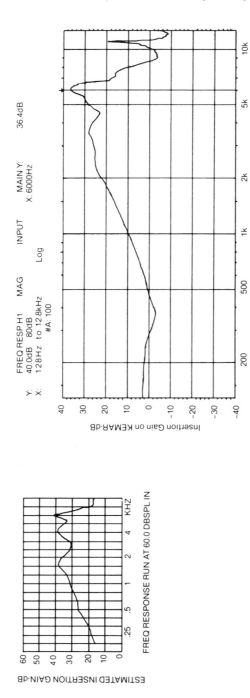

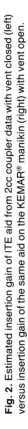

Fig. 2. Estimated insertion gain of ITE aid from 2cc coupler data with vent closed (left) versus insertion gain of the same aid on the KEMAR® manikin (right) with vent open.

by a hearing aid receiver for some individual ear canals among the 11 ears studied (Sachs and Burkhard, 1972). This can result in differences in SPL produced by the same hearing aid in different ear canals of up to 15 dB.

The differences form the rationale for *in situ* real ear measurements of hearing aid performance on an individual basis.

IN SITU ELECTROACOUSTIC MEASUREMENT OF HEARING AID PERFORMANCE

The concept of *in situ* hearing aid assessment dates back to the earliest days of hearing aid measurements (Romanow, 1942; Nichols, 1947). The term *in situ* means that measurement of hearing aid performance is performed while the hearing aid is ''on site'' or as worn. The *in situ* frequency response of a hearing aid is the output sound pressure level produced by that hearing aid in an ear canal across the frequency range of interest while that aid is being worn.

Some of the first studies of the resonance and diffraction effects produced by the human head and torso in a sound field and the resulting sound pressure produced in unaided human ear canals were made in an anechoic chamber by using a metal probe tube attached to an external microphone. The presence of this probe tube in the external auditory meatus did not significantly distort the sound field there (Wiener and Ross, 1946; Wiener, 1947). Some of the first *in situ* measurements of hearing aid performance were performed with metal probe tubes attached to laboratory-grade condenser microphones to assess the effects of varying earmold parameters such as vent diameter and canal bore length (Ewertsen et al., 1957; McDonald and Studebaker, 1970).

THE CONCEPT OF THE REAL EAR MEASUREMENT OF INSERTION GAIN

The insertion gain may be obtained by subtracting the unaided frequency response of the hearing aid wearer (wearer frequency response or WFR) from the *in situ* gain of the hearing aid.

The *in situ* gain has been defined for a manikin such as the KEMAR® manikin in ANSI standard S3.35-1985 as ''the difference between the sound pressure level (SPL) produced by the hearing aid in the manikin ear simulator and the reference sound pressure level.'' This difference is automatically obtained with the substitution method of sound field equalization. Note that the *in situ* gain of a hearing aid contains not only the output sound pressure produced by the hearing aid, but also the ''frequency response'' of the manikin (or person for real ear measurements). Thus, the *in situ* gain measurement should be used with caution because it is an overestimation of the actual *assistance* provided by a hearing aid to a hearing aid wearer in terms of improved hearing threshold levels. A valid *in situ* gain may theoretically only be determined by the substitution method of sound field equalization. Please refer to Figure 3.

The reference sound pressure level is defined in ANSI standard S3.35-1985 as ''the free-field sound pressure level at the test point in the absence of the manikin.'' Real ear probe microphone measurements are generally performed in sound field and not in the quiet, spectrally flat and. unchanging free field produced in an anechoic chamber. Consequently, because of reflections of sound off walls, the reference sound pressure level will not usually be spectrally flat over the frequency range of interest in normal everyday hearing aid evaluation test rooms or even in sound-treated industrial-grade test booths. Additionally, because of changing environmental background noise levels in the test room, the reference sound pressure level may not remain constant from measurement to measurement. It is because of these less than ideal conditions that some probe microphone systems incorporate sound field equalization methods other than the substitution method. Additionally, as later discussed, unlike the *in situ* gain

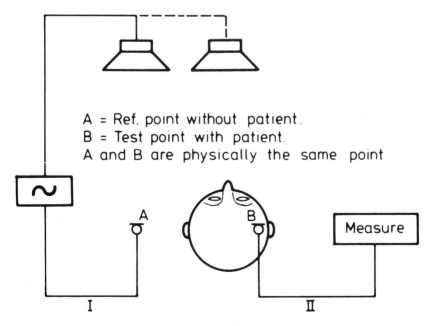

A = Ref. point without patient.
B = Test point with patient.
A and B are physically the same point

Fig. 3. Procedure for the *in situ* gain measurement with the substitution method of sound field equalization (From Madsen, 1986; Reprinted with permission)

measurement, the insertion gain measurement can be made validly with sound field equalization methods other than the substitution method. Some of the sound field equalization methods utilized by several available probe microphone systems are shown in Table 1.

Nevertheless, taking the ANSI S3.35 definitions of *in situ* gain, insertion gain and reference SPL, if "wearer" is substituted for "manikin", and "ear canal" is substituted for "manikin ear simulator", we can apply these same definitions to probe microphone measurements in real ears (Preves and Sullivan, 1987).

An insertion gain measurement will produce a lower gain figure than an *in situ* gain measurement because the unaided gain of the manikin (MFR) or hearing aid wearer (WFR) is subtracted out. The insertion gain provides an electroacoustic estimate of the functional gain, the psychoacoustic measurement obtained with an audiometer of the amount by which a hearing aid changes hearing threshold levels, relative to the unaided condition.

Some of the earliest measurements of *in situ* gain and insertion gain were performed by researchers on manikins such as KEMAR® (Knowles Electronics, 1973). For an *in situ* gain or an insertion gain measurement of a hearing aid on the KEMAR® manikin, the 1/2″ condenser microphone in a Zwislocki ear simulator serves as both the eardrum and the point at which the aided output of a hearing aid is measured. Since the KEMAR® manikin was designed to replicate a median person, the insertion gain provided by a hearing aid on the KEMAR® manikin has been shown to correlate closely with the *median* functional gain provided by that same hearing aid on a number of hearing aid wearers (Causey and Beck, 1976).

Because of the danger of injury, insertion gain measurements for real ears with probe-tube microphones are not generally performed at the eardrum but at a point between the tip of the earmold and the eardrum. As will be discussed later in this chapter, the exact placement of the probe tube in the ear canal is somewhat critical for making viable insertion gain measurements at some frequencies.

USING PROBE MICROPHONE SYSTEMS TO VERIFY PRESCRIPTIVE HEARING AID FITTINGS

One of the steps in fitting hearing aids with POGO and other prescriptive methods is verification of the acoustical performance to account for all of the inter-subject variability of the hearing aid and earmold interacting with the unique physiology of the hearing aid wearer. An example of such a verification is shown in Figure 4a: the heavy line on the right side of the figure is the desired insertion gain

Table 1.
Currently available probe microphone measurement systems and their methods of sound field equalization per ANSI and IEC documents

Device	Pressure	(Modified Comparison)	Comparison	Substitution	Equivalent Substitution	Constant Ear Canal SPL
Rastronics CCI-10 CCI-10/3	avail 2-1-87	X X		avail 1-1-87	avail 2-1-87	avail 2-1-87
Madsen IGO 1000		X		X	X	X
*AND/OR Acoustimed HA-2000				X*	X*	X*
Bosch Eartron Invivo		X				
*Frye 6500				X*	X*	X*
Biologic	X	X		X	X	X
Phonic Ear		X				
Bruel and Kjaer				X	X	X

*these systems utilize complex stimuli and do not actually equalize the input signal frequency by frequency prescribed by POGO, determined by the computer in the probe microphone system after entering the patient's audiometric hearing threshold levels. The lighter line below is the insertion gain obtained with an in-the-ear hearing on that person at the highest volume control setting possible before onset of acoustical feedback oscillation. Note that the hearing aid performs to the POGO prescription closely in the mid frequencies but has inadequate gain in the high and low frequencies. Figure 4b shows the frequency response of this hearing aid on the HA-1 2cc coupler. This hearing aid could be adjusted via frequency response trimmer potentiometers (if included) or returned to the factory for modification to achieve a closer match to the POGO prescription. In the left side of Figure 4a, the upper line is the *in situ* frequency response of the hearing aid on the wearer and the lower line is the unaided frequency response of the wearer (WFR). The difference between these two lines is the insertion gain, which is automatically plotted by the probe microphone system at the right.

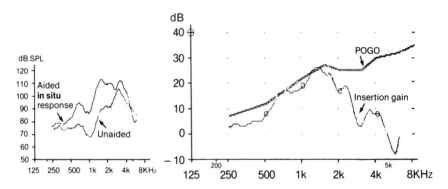

Fig. 4a. Verification of a hearing aid fitting by comparing the predicted insertion gain from POGO versus the actual insertion gain measured on the hearing aid wearer.

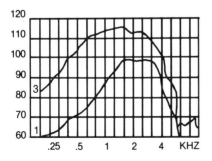

MPO CURVE(3) RUN AT 90 DBSPL INPUT

MPO = 115 0 DBSPL @ 1.600 KHZ

HFA SSPL90 = 113.3 DBSPL (IRTS = 96.3)

REF TEST GAIN = 34.0 DB

HFA FULL ON GAIN = 34.2 DB @ 60 DB IN

FREQ RESPONSE(1) RUN AT 60 DBSPL IN

F1(LF) = .590 KHZ, F2(HF) = 5.33 KHZ

Fig. 4b. 2 cc coupler data for same hearing aid.

Other hearing aid prescriptive techniques utilize most comfortable level and loudness discomfort level, in addition to or instead of hearing threshold levels for selecting the electroacoustic performance of hearing aids (Wallenfels, 1967; Victoreen, 1973; Shapiro, 1976; Pascoe, 1978). As a tool for verifying these prescriptions, some probe microphone systems have features suitable for determining hearing threshold levels, most comfortable listening level (MCL) and loudness discomfort level (LDL). These parameters would be determined in sound field using the probe microphone system loudspeaker as the sound source and the probe tube in the ear canal to sense the sound pressure level at which a particular subjective response was elicited. In order to validate this type of prescription, the probe microphone system should be capable of generating appropriate stimuli that are suitable for determining MCL and LDL, both by frequency and for complex sounds. Some probe microphone systems can generate a broad-band noise stimulus with a speech-weighted spectrum. Additionally, following the protocol suggested by Pascoe, if the probe microphone system has narrow band filters, it would be possible, for example, by using this speech noise stimulus, to verify (predict) at the common audiometric frequencies whether all components of speech, as processed by the hearing aid, would be above threshold and near MCL, but below LDL for a particular hearing aid wearer. In this application, the probe microphone system would be used to assess how much gain was supplied by the hearing aid to raise the level of the speech spectrum. One would simply measure the sound pressure level of the amplified speech spectrum noise at the hearing aid output at a particular frequency in the ear canal of a hearing aid wearer and compare that level to threshold, MCL and LDL at that same frequency. These measurements would all be performed using SPL, rather than HL, as the scale of measurement.

More accurate values can be expected from directly measuring the dB SPL at threshold, MCL and LDL is an individual real ear, as opposed to reading the values of dB HL from the attenuater of an audiometer which utilizes a headphone that has been calibrated on an NBS 9A coupler. That is, there may be significant differences between the nominal SPL calibration values on the NBS 9A coupler at a particular audiometer HL setting and the actual SPL produced by that audiometer in an individual real ear at the same setting (Hagen and Preves, 1982).

CORRELATING COMPLAINTS OF THE HEARING WEARER TO ELECTROACOUSTIC PERFORMANCE

One of the most useful applications of probe microphone systems is in predicting what electroacoustic changes in hearing aid performance would bring about solutions to hearing aid wearers' complaints. Take, for example, the insertion gain frequency response shown in Figure 4a for an ITE aid, as measured with a probe microphone system in the ear canal of the person it was designed for. It is obvious from this curve that the wearer was getting insufficient high frequency gain from this hearing aid when comparing the insertion gain response to the POGO insertion gain prescription. This particular hearing aid wearer was a chronic complainer who had been trying various hearing aids for 10 years. The poor high frequency insertion gain shown by the probe microphone correlated with the complaints of this hearing aid wearer who was unable to understand what his wife was saying very well while wearing the aid. The corresponding 2cc coupler frequency response for the ITE aid is shown in Figure 4b. The hearing aid was then returned to the manufacturer for modification. The first changes at the factory were to replace the standard response receiver with an extended high frequency response receiver and to drill out a deep bell making a stepped bore for the receiver outlet (Preves, 1980). The resulting change in the frequency response in the 2cc coupler is shown in Figure 4c. Note the increase in high frequency gain that was achieved. However, the response also became more peaky. The final change at the factory was to insert an acoustic resistance damper in the receiver tubing outlet. The result, as measured in the 2cc coupler, shown in Figure 4d is to smooth the frequency response and to give it even more high frequency gain. Thereafter, the hearing aid was tried again on the patient with the resulting insertion gain determined with probe microphone as shown in Figure 4e. Note that the insertion gain at 4kHz has increased by 10dB, as compared to that in Figure 4a, from the changes made to the ITE aid by the manufacturer. However, the required gain predicted by POGO at 4kHz is still about 10 dB greater than the hearing aid produced. It is thought from this example that POGO may predict too much high frequency gain. The formerly

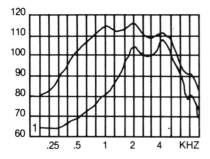

MPO CURVE(3) RUN AT 90 DBSPL INPUT
MPO = 116 6 DBSPL @ 2 000 KHZ

HFA SSPL90 = 113.6 DBSPL (IRTS = 96.6)

REF TEST GAIN = 32.0 DB
HFA FULL ON GAIN = 32.2 DB @ 60 DB IN

FREQ RESPONSE(1) RUN AT 60 DBSPL IN
F1(LF) = 600 KHZ, F2(HF) = 9.476 KHZ

Fig. 4c. 2 cc coupler data for same hearing aid after modification with an extended range receiver and a stepped bore ear canal.

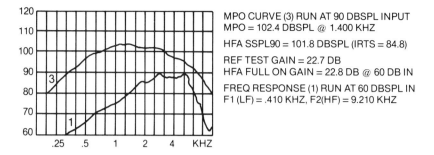

MPO CURVE (3) RUN AT 90 DBSPL INPUT
MPO = 102.4 DBSPL @ 1.400 KHZ
HFA SSPL90 = 101.8 DBSPL (IRTS = 84.8)
REF TEST GAIN = 22.7 DB
HFA FULL ON GAIN = 22.8 DB @ 60 DB IN
FREQ RESPONSE (1) RUN AT 60 DBSPL IN
F1 (LF) = .410 KHZ, F2(HF) = 9.210 KHZ

Fig. 4d. 2 cc coupler data for same hearing aid as is Figure 4c after adding an acoustic resistance damper in the receiver tubing.

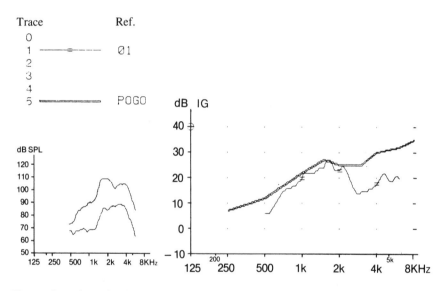

Fig. 4e. Insertion gain obtained with modified hearing aid in Figure 4d on the hearing aid wearer versus the desired POGO prescription.

chronic complaining hearing aid wearer reported highly improved listening results and has not been heard from since but must be happy since he is sending referrals to the hearing aid dispenser.

GENERAL PROCEDURES FOR UTILIZING PROBE MICROPHONE SYSTEMS

Regardless of which probe microphone system is employed, there are certain decisions and procedural steps common to insertion gain measurements. The menu system of the Madsen IGO-1000 will be referred to in this discussion (Figure 5). Among the decisions to be made and procedures to be followed are:

1. *Selection of the test type — in situ gain or insertion gain*
   If the focus of interest is the total output SPL of the hearing aid in the hearing aid wearer's ear, choose *in situ* gain; if the actual benefit provided by the hearing aid in terms of improving hearing thresholds is of interest, choose insertion gain.

2. *Selection of the stimulus type*
   If there is a choice, select the type of input stimulus to use — pure tones, warble tones, narrow band noise, wide band noise, clicks, speech, etc.

   a. Swept pure tones — can be susceptible to standing waves produced from reflections off walls in the test room and in the ear canal. This can produce lack of repeatability in the measurements if the subject or probe tube moves during the testing.

   b. Swept warble tones and narrow-band noise — better than pure tones for the standing wave subject movement and probe tube movement problems.

   c. Complex input stimuli — more representatives of the type of input hearing aids are required to process. Caution is advised since too high an input level can easily saturate the aid.

Parameters	Choices
TEST TYPE	Insertion/In Situ
STIM. TRANSMISSION	Free Field/Tele Coil
STIM. TYPE	Warble/Tone/NB Noise/Speech
PRESCRIPTION METHOD	POGO/Your own/Direct
UNOCCLUDED EAR TEST	Measure/KEMAR
TEST METHOD	Pressure/Substitution/ Ipsilateral Comparison
TEST LEVEL (SPL)	60dB/70dB/80dB
MAX. SPL AT EAR DRUM	100dB/110dB/120dB/130dB/Off
STIM. LEVEL ACCURACY	1dB/2dB/4dB
TEST SAMPLES	12/24/48 per Octave
FREQ. RANGE LOWER LIMIT	125Hz/250Hz/500Hz
FREQ. RANGE UPPER LIMIT	4000Hz/6000Hz/8000Hz
FACTORY DEFAULT PROGRAM	No/Yes
SAVE PROGRAM	Yes/No

Fig. 5. Usage of menus in Madsen IGO-1000 probe microphone system. (Reprinted with permission.)

     i. Clicks — like broadband noise but with controlled phase; too high an input level can easily overload hearing aids.

    ii. Random noise — like white noise from an audiometer; having no control of the noise peaks can easily saturate hearing aids when too great an input level is used.

   iii. Pseudo random noise — like random noise but digitally generated with controlled phase to regulate peak energy.

   iv. Speech — the input stimulus of interest in real world use of a hearing aid. Harder to reproduce at a given instant in time than most other input stimuli.

3. *Selection of the sound field equalization method.*
If there is a choice, decide which method of sound field equalization to use — substitution, pressure, comparison, etc. Some probe microphone systems such as the Madsen IGO-1000 employ more than one sound field equalization method and allow the operator to select. For *in situ* gain measurements, theoretically only the substitution method is appropriate in order to include all of the effects of the hearing aid wearer's body. For measurement of insertion gain, most sound field equalization methods should work equally well if the operator carefully observes certain precautions.

4. *Selection of the input level*
If there is a choice, select the input level of the particular test stimulus selected with caution as per the above comments. Generally, the lower the input level, the greater the chances that noise in the test environment will affect the results. However, too high an input level such as 80 dB SPL or even 70 dB SPL with a swept pure tone, warble tone or narrow band noise may saturate the hearing aid and produce artificially flatened frequency responses. Normally, 60 dB SPL is a good input level for swept pure tones, warble tones and narrow band noise. However, 50 dB SPL may be required for broad band noise and clicks in order to keep the aid out of saturation.

5. *Selection of the frequency resolution*
If there is a choice, select the number of test frequencies to be utilized within the frequency range. Generally, the greater the number of test frequencies, the smoother and more accurate the response curve is, but at the expense of longer test time.

6. *Selection of the frequency range*
If there is a choice, select the upper and lower frequency limits at which the system will test. For example, if a hearing aid having a

large vent in the earmold is not expected to have much real ear gain below 500 Hz, then 500 Hz would be a good lower limit test frequency. Correspondingly, if fitting a ski-slope audiometric configuration and the high frequency gain is of interest, 6000 Hz or 8000 Hz may be a good upper limit test frequency. Generally, but not always, a wider frequency range may require longer test time.

PATIENT MOVEMENT AND PROBE MICROPHONE PLACEMENT PROBLEMS

It is well known that due to standing waves in the test booth, any physical movement of a hearing aid wearer's body during audiometric sound field assessments of functional gain can result in invalid data. Similarly, any movement of a patient during probe microphone measurements of insertion gain can result in invalid data 1) if the input sound pressure at the location of the hearing aid microphone changes between unaided and aided measurements or 2) if the location of the tip of the probe tube in the ear canal changes between unaided and aided measurements. Both problems can be minimized by using a dental chair type headrest to provide increased comfort for the patient and help immobilize the patient's head during the insertion gain measurements.

The exact location of the probe microphone in the ear canal is not particularly critical for frequencies below 4kHz if it does not move between unaided and aided measurements (Preves, 1984). At higher frequencies, standing waves in the ear canal can allow probe movement between measurements to provide erroneous data if the tip of the probe tube is placed further out in the ear canal than about 3/8″ from the eardrum (Figure 6). Note, for example, in this figure, at a relative probe position of 4/8″, deviations of the sound pressure level from that very near the eardrum are −20dB for 6kHz and −8 dB for 4kHz due to standing waves. However, at the same position, there is no problem at 1kHz and at 2kHz.

There is also a problem of encountering a drop in sound pressure with a pure tone input stimulus if the tip of the probe tube is placed too near the earmold outlet (Sachs and Burkhard, 1977). As the sound emanates from the small hole in the earmold and spreads to the larger residual ear canal volume, the SPL drops to a minimum at higher frequencies at close distances from the tip of the earmold. Keeping the end of the probe tube at least 4 mm beyond the tip of the earmold will keep this from being a problem.

In any case, accuracy of probe tube placement is enhanced by using a otoscope or an ear light. Additionally, some probe tubes have cylindrical rings on them which can be moved up and down the probe tube to form a reference point for probe tube depth.

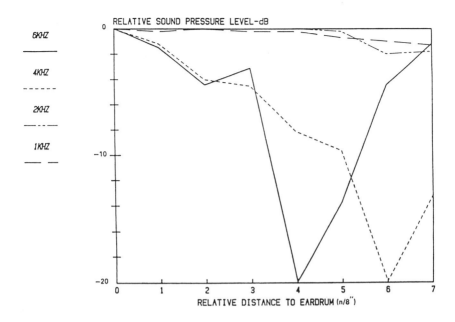

Fig. 6. Effect of probe depth in the KEMAR® manikin ear canal at 4 frequencies. Deviation of SPL shown from position near "eardrum". (Reprinted with permission).

DESIRABLE FEATURES FOR PROBE MICROPHONE SYSTEMS

Since most of the available probe microphone systems are microprocessor-based, one would excpect them to have at least some of the capabilities found in popular personal computers. These include:

— a conventional microcomputer typewriter-like keyboard

— a menu-driven command structure so that key strokes do not have to be memorized to perform commands

— a graphics video terminal (CRT) — color preferred-for viewing both the menus and the frequency responses derived

— capability of storing, recalling and erasing data via disk

The more these features are included in a probe microphone system, the more powerful the system will probably be because its capability can continually be upgraded by software changes. It can also be used for other traditional microcomputer applications such as word processing, accounting and data base patient record keeping. Pictures of representative probe microphone systems are shown in Figures 7, 8, 9, 10 and 11.

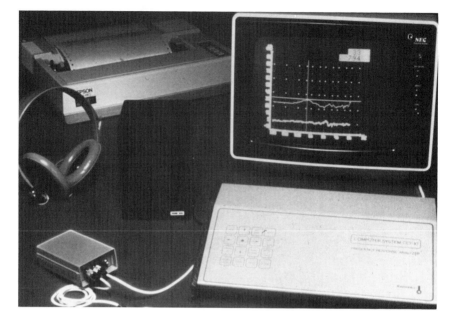

Fig. 7. Rastronics CCI-10/3 (Reprinted with permission)

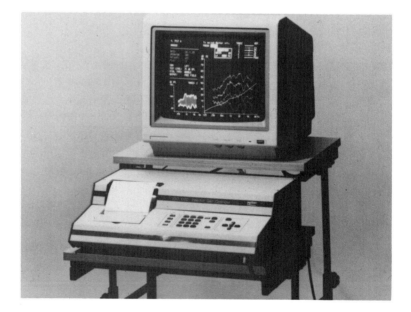

Fig. 8. Madsen IGO-1000A probe microphone system. The straight line on the screen is the desired insertion gain predicted by the POGO method. (Reprinted with permission.)

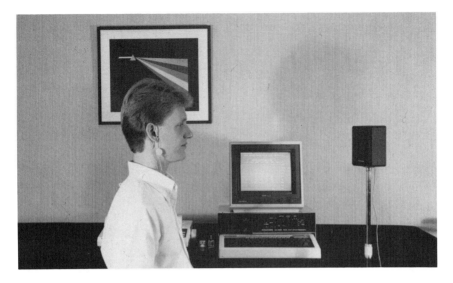

Fig. 9. Acoustimed HA-2000 probe microphone system. (Reprinted with permission from And/Or Corp.)

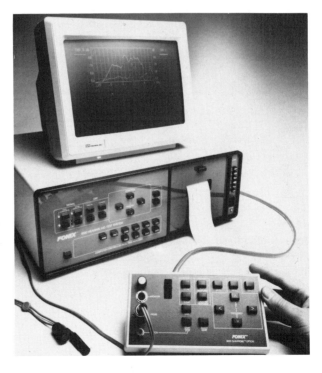

Fig. 10. Frye 6500 probe microphone system. (Reprinted with permission.)

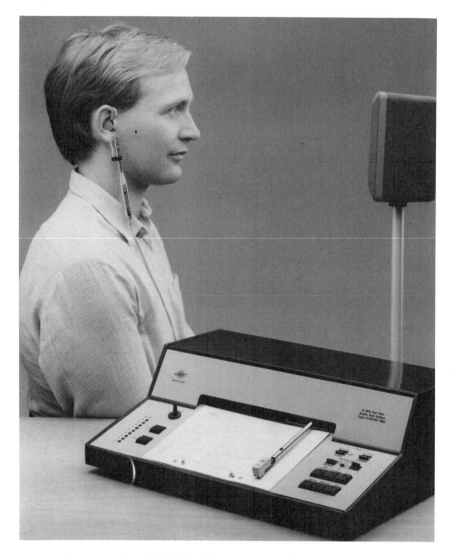

Fig. 11. Bruel and Kjaer 2118/WH 1823 probe microphone system. (Reprinted with permission.)

Additionally, the probe microphone system should be capable of:

— subtracting two frequency responses

— rapidly measuring either insertion gain or *in situ* gain

— providing variable input levels

- providing a choice of wide band (complex) and narrow band input stimuli
- having enough test frequencies for drawing smooth responses
- a method for directly calibrating the reference microphone
- providing an easy method of starting over during an automatic test sequence without starting the program from the very beginning
- physically separating the reference microphone from the probe-tube microphone if two microphones are used for greatest flexibility and measurement validity
- providing the substitution equalization method to conform to the methods outlined in ANSI S3.35-1985 for measuring *in situ* gain.
- performing 2cc coupler measurements per ANSI S3.22-1982

Salient features of some available probe microphone systems are shown in Table 2.

Table 2.
Available Probe Microphone Systems Versus Salient Features

System	CRT	Subtracts Curves	Substitution Equalization	Full Keyboard	Disk Store	Complex Input
Rastronics CCI-10/3	Y	Y	N	N	N	Y
Madsen IGO 1000	Y	Y	Y	N	N	N
Acoustimed HA-2000	Y	Y	Y*	Y	Y	Y
*Frye 6500	Y	Y	Y*	N	N	Y
Bruel & Kjaer 2118/ WH 1823	N	Y	Y	N	N	N
Horag Eartron Invivo	N	N	N	N	N	N
Biologic Systems	Y	Y	Y	Y	Y	Y
Phonic Ear	N	N	N	N	N	N

*does not actually equalize the input stimulus, frequency by frequency

SUMMARY

Probe microphone systems may be used to validate hearing aid fittings prescribed in accordance with a wide variety of prescription hearing aid fitting techniques. For those prescriptive techniques that utilize functional gain for validation, the real ear measurement of insertion gain, as determined with a probe microphone system, may be effectively used as an approximation of the functional gain provided by a hearing aid on an individual basis. Because probe microphone systems can measure sound pressure levels in a hearing aid wearer's ear canal, these systems may also be used to determine hearing threshold levels, most comfortable listening levels and loudness discomfort levels on an individual basis. Some of the microcomputer-based probe microphone systems have the capability of calculating the desired electroacoustic response of a hearing aid fitting from audiological data with an extensive selection of prescriptive methods.

There can be problems in obtaining valid probe microphone data unless the operator understands the options and tradeoffs in selecting a sound field equalization method, the type of input stimulus and the input level, among other variables. Erroneous data can result unless certain procedures for probe tube and subject placement are carefully followed.

Hopefully, this chapter will be of assistance in applying probe microphone systems to validate hearing aid fittings.

GLOSSARY

Anechoic chamber: A sound-proofed enclosure which contains acoustically absorbent material on its inner surfaces to attenuate external sounds and to prevent reverberation.

Bit: Standing for binary digit and the numerical basis of all digital computers; a digit based on the binary number system which takes value of "1" or "0".

Byte: A string of several bits making up a "word" as used by a digital computer; frequently refers to computer memory.

CRT: Abbreviation for cathode ray tube; a monitor similar to a television screen with which to view computer selection menus, keyboard entries and data obtained and recalled.

Disk: A flat rotating magnetic surface used for storing data; "floppy" disks are usually either 3-1/2" or 5-1/4" square and can store up to 1.2 megabytes of data; "hard" disks can store up to 100 megabytes of data.

Electroacoustic measure: Referring to a physical measurement of a hearing aid output in which no behavioral response is required from the hearing aid wearer being evaluated. e.g. insertion gain.

Equalization: Referring to removing the variations in amplitude of an input sound field produced by a loudspeaker over the frequency range of interest.

EEE: Abbreviation for external ear effects; the unaided frequency response as measured in a human ear canal using the pressure method of sound field equalization (Sullivan, 1985).

Free field: The radiation produced by a loudspeaker in an anechoic environment.

Free field environment: An environment totally free of reverberation from nearby surfaces; e.g. an anechoic chamber.

Functional gain: A psychoacoustic measurement of the difference, as determined with an audiometer at discrete frequencies, that is produced by a hearing aid on a hearing impaired person between the unaided and the aided hearing threshold levels.

Insertion gain: An electroacoustic measurement of the difference between the unaided and aided sound pressure levels that are produced by a hearing aid in an ear canal, as determined with a probe tube microphone system at discrete frequencies.

In situ: A latin phrase standing for on site.

In situ gain: The difference between the output sound pressure level produced by a hearing aid in an ear canal and the sound pressure level at the same location within the test environment but without the hearing aid wearer present. Strictly speaking, only the substitution method of equalization procudes a valid *in situ* gain measurement.

KEMAR: Abbreviation for Knowles Electronics Manikin for Acoustic Research; a human-like device with dimensions determined from the average of 5200 males and females; suitable for making measurements of hearing aids *in situ*.

Keyboard: A set of keys like those on a typewriter with which to enter commands and patient and data labelling information to a microcomputer.

MFR: Abbreviation for manikin frequency response; the unaided frequency response of a manikin as measured using the substitution method of equalization.

Menu: A group of selectable commands displayed on a computer monitor screen.

Monitor: A screen like a television for viewing computer keyboard entries, data obtained and recalled and selection menus.

POGO: Abbreviation for prescription of gain and output; a hearing aid prescription method based on the real ear measurement of insertion gain.

Prescription method: A means of predicting the electroacoustic performance of a hearing aid from audiological and patient history data.

Probe tube: A narrow diameter flexible tube, designed to extend in to human ear canals, one end of which attaches to a microphone while the other end remains open to allow sounds to enter.

Probe tube microphone: A microphone which has a narrow diameter tube attached to its inlet for picking up sounds in human ear canals.

Psychoacoustic measure: Referring to a behavioral measure requiring a response from the hearing aid wearer being evaluated; e.g. functional gain.

Reference sound pressure level: A base line from which to compare the output of a hearing aid; e.g. the input to a hearing aid in a sound chamber or, for real ear measurements, the sound pressure level at the test point in the absence of the hearing aid wearer.

Reference microphone: A microphone which monitors the input sound pressure to the hearing aid; is often used in a compressor loop to keep the input sound pressure level constant at a particular location.

ROM: Abbreviation for read only memory; a means of storing programs for a computer with semiconductor integrated circuits.

Sound field: The radiation produced by a loudspeaker in a non-anechoic environment.

Sound field environment: An environment which is not a free field because some reflections are present from nearby surfaces; e.g. a sound-treated room.

Substitution method: The sound field equalization method defined in ANSI standard S3.35-1985 for making simulated real measurements of hearing aid performance on a manikin. This method can be adapted for real ear measurements and results in the determination of *in situ* gain by including the total diffraction effects of the hearing aid wearer's body in the real ear output of the aid.

Test point: The physical location in the testing environment at the center of the hearing aid wearer's head.

WFR: Abbreviation for wearer frequency response; the unaided frequency response of a human as measured in a human ear canal utilizing the substitution method of equalization (Preves and Sullivan, 1987).

REFERENCES

ANSI (American National Standards Institute): Methods of measurement of performance characteristics of hearing aids under simulated *in situ* working conditions, S3.35-1985, 8-9, 1985.

ARLINGER, S. and JERLVALL, L.: Measurement of hearing aid real ear gain: a comparison between the miniature microphone and the hearing threshold methods, paper pres. at Current Topics in Audiology conf., Irvine, California, August 23-24, 1984.

AYERS, E.: A discussion of some problems involved in deriving objective performance criteria for a wearable hearing aid from clinical measurements with laboratory apparatus, Proc. of 1st ICA Congress, Delft, 141-143, 1953.

BERANEK, L.: *Acoustic Measurement,* Wiley, N.Y., 1949.

BERGER, K.: Prescription of hearing aids, a rationale, Kent State University, 1976.

BROOKS, D.: Gain requirements of hearing aid users, Scand. Audiol., 2, 4, 199-205, 1973.

BURKHARD, M. and SACHS, R.: Sound pressure in insert earphone couplers and real ears, J. Speech Hear. Res., 20, 799-807, 1977.

BYRNE, D. and TONNISON, W.: Selecting the gain of hearing aids for persons with sensorineural hearing impairments, Scand. Audiol., 5, 51-69, 1976.

BYRNE, D. and DILLON, H.: The National Acoustic Laboratories' (NAL) new procedure for selecting the gain and frequency response of a hearing aid, Ear and Hearing, 7, 4, 257-265, 1986.

CAUSEY, G. D. and BECK, L.: Relationship of measurements on KEMAR to behavioral performance, paper pres. at 13th Int'l Congress of Audiol., Florence, Italy, 1976.

COX, R.: A structured approach to hearing aid selection, Ear and Hearing, 6, 5, 226-239, 1985.

DAHLSGAARD, S. and JENSEN, O.: Measurements of the insertion gain of hearing aids. J. Audiol. Tech. 15, 170-183, 1976.

DAHLSGAARD, S., JOHANSEN, P. and CHISNALL, L.: On the frequency response of ear-moulds, J. Audiol. Tech., 5(4), 126-139, 1966.

DILLON, H. and MURRAY, N.: Accuracy of twelve methods of estimating the real ear gain of hearing aids, Ear and Hearing, 8, 1, 1987.

EWERTSEN, H., IPSEN, J., and NIELSEN, S.: On acoustical characteristics of the earmold, Acta Otolaryngolica, 47, 312-317, 1957.

HAGEN, L. and PREVES, D.: Beyond the NBS-9A coupler: the probe microphone as an SPL determinant, Hear. J., 35, 8, 7-12, 1982.

HARFORD, E.: The use of real ear measures for fitting wearable amplification, Hear J., 7, 1, 1984.

DE JONGE, R.: Users Manual for Select an Aid, 1985.

KILLION, M.: personal communication, 1986.

KNOWLES ELECTRONICS: KEMAR the Knowles Electronics Manikin for Acoustic Research, Report No. 20032-1, 1973.

LIBBY, E.: State-of-the-art of hearing aid selection procedures, Hear. Inst., 36, 1, 30-38.

LYBARGER, S.: U.S. Patent Application 543, 278, 1944.

LYBARGER, S.: *Simplified Fitting System for Hearing Aids,* Radioear Specifications and fitting information manual, 1-8, Oct., 1963.

LYBARGER, S. and TEDER, H.: 2 cc coupler curves to insertion gain curves: calculated and experimental results, Hear. Inst., 37, 11, 36-40, 1986.

MADSEN, P.: Insertion gain optimization, Hear. Inst., 37, 1, 28-32, 1986.

MARKLE, D. and ZANER, A.: The determination of "gain requirements" of hearing aids: a new method, J. of Auditory Research, 6, 371-377, 1966.

MARTIN, M.: Hearing aid gain requirements in sensorineural hearing loss, Brit. J. of Audiol., 7, 21-24, 1973.

MASON, D. and POPELKA, G.: A Users Guide for Phase IV Hearing Aid Selection and Evaluation Program, version 1.1b, Central Inst. for the Deaf, St. Louis, MO, 1982.

McCANDLESS, G. and LYREGAARD, P.: Prescription of gain/output (POGO) for hearing aids, Hear. Inst., 34, 1:16-21, 1983.

McDONALD, F. and STUDEBAKER, G: Earmold alteration effects as measured in the human auditory meatus, J. Acoust. Soc. Am., 22(5), 329-334, 1970.

MILLIN, J.: Speech discrimination as a function of hearing aid gain, Implications in hearing aid evaluation, Masters Thesis, Western Reserve Univ., Cleveland, OH, 1965.

NICHOLS, R.: The influence of body-baffle effects on the performance of hearing aids, J. Acoust. Soc. of Amer., 19, 943, 1947.

OLSSON, ULF: Hearing aid measurements on occluded-ear simulator compared to simulated *in situ* and *in situ* measurements, Report TA111, Karolinska Instit. Dept. of Technical Audiology, Stockkholm, Sweden, 1985.

PASCOE, D.: Frequency responses of hearing aids and their effects on the speech perception of hearing impaired subjects, Annals of Oto., Rhino., and Laryn. Supp., 23, 84, 5, 2, 1975.

PASCOE, D.: An approach to hearing aid selection, Hearing Inst., 29, 6, 12-13, 1978.

PREVES, D.: Effects of earmold venting on coupler, manikin, and real ears, Hear. Aid J., 30, 43-46, 1977.

PREVES, D.: Stepped bore earmolds for custom ITE hearing aids, Hear. Inst., 31, 10, 24-26, 1980.

PREVES, D.: Levels of realism in hearing aid measurement techniques, Hear J., 37, 7, 13-19, 1984.

PREVES, D. and ORTON, J.: Use of acoustic impedance measures in hearing aid fitting, Hearing Inst., 29, 6, 22-24, 34, 1978.

PREVES, D. and SULLIVAN, R.: Methods of sound field equalization for real ear measurements with probe microphones, Hear. Inst., 38, 1, 20-26, 1987.

REDDELL, R. and CALVERT, D.: Selecting a hearing aid by interpreting audiologic data, J. of Auditory Research, 6, 445-452, 1966.

ROMANOV, F.: Methods for measuring the performance of hearing aids, J. Acoust. Soc. of Am., 13, 294-304, 1942.

RUMOSHOSKY, J. and PREVES, D.: Hearing aid evaluations using custom in-the-ear and stock behind-the-ear aids, Hearing Aid J., 30, 10, 11, 46-49, 1976.

SCHWARTZ, D.: Hearing aid selection methods: an enigma, *The Vanderbilt Report,* ed. Studebaker, G. and Bess, F., Upper Darby, PA, 180-187, 1982.

SHORE, I., BILGER, R., and HIRSCH, I.: Hearing aid evaluation: reliability of repeated measurements, J. Speech and Hear. Disorders, 25, 152-170, 1960.

SEILER, J.: A formula for fitting hearing aids, Hearing Dealer, 22. 18-19, 1971.

SHAPIRO, I.: Hearing aid fitting by prescription, Audiology, 15, 163-173, 1976.

SKINNER, M., PASCOE, D., MILLER, J., POPELKA, G.: (Measurements to determine the optimal placement of speech energy within the listener's auditory area: a basis of selecting amplification characteristics, *The Vanderbilt Report,* ed. Studebaker, G. and Bess, F., Upper Darby, PA, 161-169, 1982.

STUDEBAKER, G.: Hearing aid selection: and overview, *The Vanderbilt Report,* ed. Studebaker, G. and Bess, F., Upper Darby, PA, 147-155, 1982.

SULLIVAN, R.: An acoustic coupling-based classification system for hearing aid fittings, Part I, Hearing Inst., 36, 9, 25-28, 1985.

TECCA, J. and WOODFORD, C.: A comparison and functional gain and insertion gain, Paper pres. at Amer. Speech and Hearing Conv., Washington, D.C., 1985.

THORNTON, A. and RAFFIN, M.: Speech-discrimination scores modeled as a binominal variable, J. Speech and Hear. Res., 21, 507-581, 1978.

VICTOREEN, J.: *Basic Principles of Otometry,* Thomas, Springfield, IL, 1973.

WALLENFELS, H.: *Hearing Aids on Prescription,* Thomas, Springfield, IL, 1967.

WATSEN, N. and KNUTSEN, V.: Selective amplification in hearing aids, J. Acoust. Soc. of Am., 11, 406-419, 1940.

WIENER, F. and ROSS, D.: The pressure distribution in the auditory canal in a progressive sound field, J. Acoust. Soc. of Amer., 18, 2, 401-407, 1946.

WIENER, F.: On the diffraction of a progressive sound wave by the human head, J. Acoust. Soc. of Am., 19, 1, 142-146, 1947.

ZEMPLENYI, J., DIRKS, D., and GILMAN, S.: Probe-determined hearing-aid gain compared to functional and coupler gains, J. Speech and Hear. Res., 28, 394-404, 1985.

VII

SOUND FIELD AUDIOMETRY AND HEARING AID SELECTION

JOHN K. DUFFY

INTRODUCTION

Audition is a sensory experience. Auditory awareness involves the entire hearing mechanism and cannot be evaluated through electroacoustic measurements that terminate at the tympanic membrane. From a professional as well as from a practical standpoint a person's auditory recognition and perception of acoustic stimuli, transmitted through a hearing aid, can, at the present time, only be measured through soundfield audiometry.

CHAPTER OBJECTIVES

In keeping with the above title and in support of the preceding statement, this chapter includes:

1 Suggestions regarding pure tone and speech measurements of hearing as a first step in identifying persons for whom amplification seems to be indicated.

2 Considerations for selecting a hearing aid which will provide optimum amplification for speech reception and phoneme recognition. This includes electroacoustic as well as psychoacoustic measurements of hearing aid response characteristics.

3 A discussion of the significance of unaided and aided auditory responses in a soundfield to tones and speech in relation to hearing aid evaluation and advisement.

4 The function of phoneme recognition testing and THE SPEECH PERCEPTION INDEX as it relates to counseling and advisement as well as to auditory and auditory-visual learning in hearing rehabilitation.

PURE-TONE AUDIOMETRY

The professional literature has dealt generously with pure-tone audiometry, therefore, our treatment of the subject will be brief. When pure-tone audiometry determines that the client's hearing, in the frequency range most critical for understanding speech (250 Hz - 4000 Hz), falls below the limits for normal hearing (30 dB and greater) the use of a suitable hearing aid is usually indicated. Following are a few suggestions for obtaining reliable and valid hearing measurements upon which judgments regarding the use of a hearing aid can be made.

In order to avoid false positive response in audiometric testing (client responding when tone is not present) we recommend that the client be instructed to respond (raise hand or finger or press signal button) as soon as he hears the tone, to keep responding as long as the tone is heard, and, when the tone is no longer heard to stop responding immediately. Of course, the testor must vary the presentations of the tone in regard to the length of pauses between presentations and the duration of presentations. A reliable client will respond promptly when the tone is presented and discontinue the response as soon as the signal is terminated.

With the above technique the client must respond twice, when the tone is presented and when it is discontinued. No client can consistently respond correctly to the tone, thus presented, unless it is heard. The client who is given only short bursts of the tone when being tested will learn to merely flip his hand or finger up and down or momentarily press the signal button when he thinks he hears the tone. Such a response may happen to correspond to the tone presentation although the tone was not heard by the client. As a result the client may give misleading false positive responses. This often occurs with children or the elderly.

In order to determine the amplification needs of a client based upon reliable audiometric measurements the client must be taught, from the outset, to respond properly during the testing. This is also important because later the same testing procedure will be used for unaided and aided soundfield measurements.

EAR SELECTION FOR AID

For a client with a symmetrical hearing loss which is moderate (45 dB - 75 dB) or severe (75 dB or greater) binaural hearing aids should be considered unless it is found, and speech audiometry confirms, that amplification in only one ear better serves the client than would wearing hearing aids in both ears. In some clients speech perception in one ear is relatively much better than it is in the other ear. In such cases, when both ears are aided, amplification in the poorer ear often interferes with the perception of speech in the better ear.

In selecting the proper ear when only one aid is to be worn it is usually found that the ear with the better bone conduction and with the better hearing above 1000 Hz is the ear most suitable for the use of amplification. Again, this decision must be supported by properly conducted speech audiometry (Duffy 1984). (Zelnick discussed binaural hearing in Chapter II).

MULTI-FREQUENCY TESTING

Another matter to consider is the need to discover hearing sensitivity at frequencies which lie between the discrete frequencies being tested. The practice of skipping 750 Hz, 1500 Hz and sometimes 3000 Hz is unwise, especially if the difference in response between any two frequencies is 15 dB or greater. A case comes to mind where the client had a threshold of 40 dB at 1000 Hz and 75 dB at 2000 Hz. Neglecting to test 1500 Hz in this instance was inexcusable. When 1500 Hz was tested the loss was 50 dB. In testing 1800 Hz the loss was found to be 50 dB. A 25 dB drop occurred between 1800 Hz and 2000 Hz. Fortunately for the client the loss was gradual from 1000 Hz through 1800 Hz, an important part of the frequency range necessary for perceiving speech, and a hearing aid proved to be more helpful than might otherwise be expected. (See Fig. 1).

For hearing aid dispensers in the market for an audiometer I suggest that they consider one which provides for multi-frequency testing between octave points as well as one that also provides for 1 dB intensity changes. In a critical area such as in the case mentioned above a more refined threshold measurement is desirable. Also, the audiometer should have warble tone capability. Such an audiometer, used for

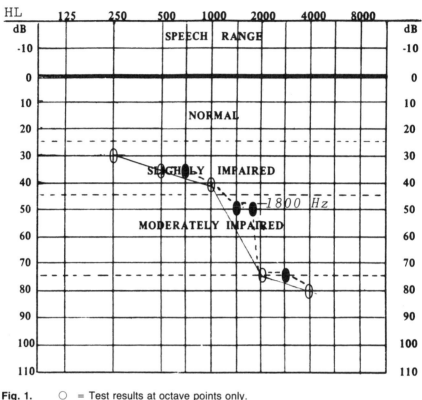

FREQUENCY IN HERTZ

Fig. 1.   ○ = Test results at octave points only.
○ – ● = Test using multi-frequency points.

head phone and soundfield measurements, will make the process of testing considerably more refined than is possible with an ordinary discrete frequency audiometer.

ORDER OF TONE PRESENTATION

The practice of starting the testing at 1000 Hz and continuing to test the frequencies above 1000 Hz in an ascending order, then, retesting 1000 Hz and testing the frequencies below 1000 Hz in descending order should be discarded for the following reasons:

    1 Because the majority of hearing-impaired persons have better hearing below 1000 Hz.

2 Because the frequencies of the audiometer, the audiogram chart, and tabular audiometric recording forms all go from low to high, it makes more sense to start the test with the lowest frequency and then to continue testing in sequential order. This method is easier, faster and more efficient than by the outmoded testing procedure that starts at 1000 Hz.

SPEECH AUDIOMETRY

Traditional speech discrimination testing using various 50 monosyllabic word lists is not a reliable procedure for providing information upon which hearing aid selection decisions can be made. For over 20 years knowledgeable professionals have known that fact. (Duffy 1967, 1978).

In conventional speech audiometry, when using the 50 monosyllabic word lists, two points of credit are assigned to each word correctly repeated. No credit is given if all but one phoneme in the word is correct as in the case of "pan" for "fan". Visual awareness of the [f] would have avoided this error in a real life situation. Because no credit is given for words partially correct, the test's score does not reflect the client's recognition of auditory cues, which, along with contextual and visual cues would contribute greatly to the client's speech perception ability. Furthermore, all that is recorded is the score. No record of the phonemes which are correct or are incorrect, are made. That such a crude testing instrument has been employed for so long is, to say the least, unfortunate.

The goal of amplification for the hearing-impaired person should be to achieve the greatest possible improvement in the ability to perceive speech. The great number of variables which influence speech comprehension in every day life make measuring the comparative effectiveness of various hearing aids possible only if we confine our evaluation to the task the hearing aid is designed to do, namely, make speech sounds audible.

Some of these variables include:

1 The kind, extent, and onset of hearing impairment.

2 Knowledge of the language spoken and the subject matter of the message.

3 The ability to utilize minimal auditory cues.

4 The ability to utilize supplementary and complementary visual cues when watching the face of the speaker.

5 Other complicating factors include: age, intelligence, attention span, health, emotional state.

Of the above variables, our concern is in providing the acoustic cues essential for the auditory perception of speech. By providing the acoustic information needed for phoneme recognition, most hearing-impaired persons will acquire improved speech perception ability. This, however, can only be accomplished with the proper use of selective amplification.

In order to discover if proper amplification is being provided by the hearing aid under test, the user's phoneme recognition must be evaluated. We have devised phoneme recognition tests which provide this information. They will be discussed later. Meanwhile, the phonemes (speech sounds) of English speech and their acoustic properties will be reviewed. This information, we trust, will make speech audiometry meaningful, practical, and useful as an instrument in hearing aid selection and evaluation and in hearing rehabilitation.

In order to identify the various speech sounds in a simple and practical manner I have devised a phonetic alphabet with letter symbols borrowed from English, The International Phonetic Alphabet and Pitman's Initial Teaching Alphabet.

This phonetic alphabet (see Table 1) is made up of letter symbols whereby each letter has been assigned a sound usually associated with that letter in many common English words. For the English letter symbols associated with different sounds in different words special symbols have been employed. Fortunately, this required only six new letter symbols which can easily be learned and associated with the phonemes they represent. English, unlike Hebrew, Italian and Russian, is not a phonetic language. In English some letter symbols represent different sounds in different words. To avoid confusion I have chosen to use my phonetic alphabet in the phoneme recognition tests and in discussing acoustic phonetics.

ACOUSTIC PHONETICS

Following is a discussion of acoustic phonetics in relation to selective amplification and speech perception.

The average range of the fundamental frequencies contained in the typical voices of children, women and men is from 124 Hz to 274 Hz according to data from research by Peterson and Barney (1952). The overtones of the fundamental frequencies, called formants, produce the acoustic characteristics that give speech sounds the distinguishing features by which we identify them. These features can be recognized even if the fundamental frequencies that produce them are inaudible to the listener.

Based upon data from Peterson and Barney (1952) Table 2 contains the ranges for the fundamental frequencies and the formants for 11 basic

**Table 1
The Phonetic Alphabet*
For
The Phoneme Recognition Inventory
and
The Phoneme Recognition Quick Test**

Vowels	Semivowels		Consonants	
[ɛ] - beat	[r] - river	**Unvoiced**		**Voiced**
[i] - bit	[l] - little	[p] - pat		[b] - bat
[æ] - bait	[w] - we	[t] - to		[d] - do
[e] - bet	[y] - you	[k]-key [c]-cat		[g] - go
[a] - bat		[f] - fan		[v] - van
[u] - but	**Diphthongs**	[th] - thin		[th] - then
[a] - far [o] - hot	[ai] - eye	[s] - see		[z] - zoo
[ɔ] - saw	[oω] - cow	[sh] - shoe		[zh] - vision
[œ] - boat	[ɔi] - boy	[ch] - chair		[j] - jar
[ω] - book		[h] - hot		[wh] - when
[ω] - boot	**Nasal Consonants**			
	[m] - man			
	[n] - no			
	[ng] - sing			

* *This phonetic alphabet, devised by John K. Duffy, is made up of the letter symbols of the regular English Alphabet, the International Phonetic Alphabet, and Pitman's Initial Teaching Alphabet. The English letter and phoneme relationship is preserved wherever possible to ease the transition from phonetic to traditional English spelling.*

vowels plus the semivowels [r] and [l]. Figure 2 is a graphic representation of this information. Note that the first and second formants for the following back vowels lie between 400 Hz and 1600 Hz: [ϑ]-boot; [ω]-book; [œ]-boat; [ɔ]-saw; [d]-father or [o]-hot; [u]-but. Hearing through this range of frequencies permits recognition of these sounds but also recognition of transitional frequencies leading to other speech sounds with second and third formants above 1600 Hz.

The second and third formants for semivowels [r] and [l] extend from 1190 Hz to 3730 Hz while the front vowels [a]-bat; [e]-bet; [æ]-bait; [i]-bit; and [ɛ]-beat; are above 1700 Hz. This means that recognition of these phonemes, in the absence of transitional cues, requires audibility which extends almost to 4000 Hz.

Besides phonemes that are produced through vocalization and have tonal characteristics, there are phonemes called unvoiced consonants that are not vocalized but are the result of air under pressure escaping as friction noise or explosive noise. These speech sounds are composed of various combinations of frequencies and are classified as fricatives (friction); plosives (explosion); affricatives (both friction and explo-

Table 2

**Frequency Spectrum of Vowels and Semivowels for
the Average Speech of Men, Women and Children***

Frequency in Hertz

Phoneme	Fundamental	First Formant	Second Formant	Third Formant
[ɛ] beat	136-272	270-3220	2290-370	3010-3730
[i] bit	135-269	390-530	1990-2730	2550-3600
[æ] bait	130-269	390-690	1840-2730	2480-3600
[e] bet	130-260	530-690	1840-2610	2480-3570
[a] bat	127-251	660-1010	1720-2320	2410-3320
[l] tell	130-261	490-850	1190-1820	1690-3360
[r] far	133-261	490-560	1350-1820	1690-2160
[u] but	130-261	640-850	1190-1590	2390-3360
[a][o]hot far	124-256	730-1030	1090-1370	2440-3170
[ɔ] saw	129-263	570-680	840-1060	2410-3180
[œ] go	130-275	440-680	840-1410	2410-3310
[ω] book	137-276	440-560	1020-1410	2240-3310
[ω] boot	141-274	300-430	870-1170	2240-3260

*Data adapted from the research of Peterson and Barney (1952)[4]
Table 2. Frequency Spectrum of Vowels and Semivowels.

sion). These phonemes are: Plosives — [p]; [t]; [k]. Fricatives — [th]; [f]; [s]; [h]; [sh]. Affricative — [ch].

The frequency composition of these unvoiced consonants is spread throughout the speech spectrum with many of the most important frequencies, for phoneme recognition, falling in the range: 1000 Hz to 4000 Hz. Some frequencies in a sharp [s] may extend as high as 7000 Hz but for recognition of the [s], in normal speech, audibility up to 4000 Hz is sufficient.

The voiced and unvoiced consonants are placed in pairs because of the similar manner in which they are produced. They differ in that one of the pair is voiced and the other is unvoiced. For example: [p] is the unvoiced cognate of [b].

Unvoiced	Voiced	Unvoiced	Voiced	Unvoiced	Voiced
p	b	f	v	sh	zh
t	d	th	th	ch	j
k(c)	g	s	z	h	wh

FREQUENCY SPECTRUM OF VOWELS AND SEMIVOWELS FOR
THE AVERAGE SPEECH OF MEN, WOMEN AND CHILDREN *

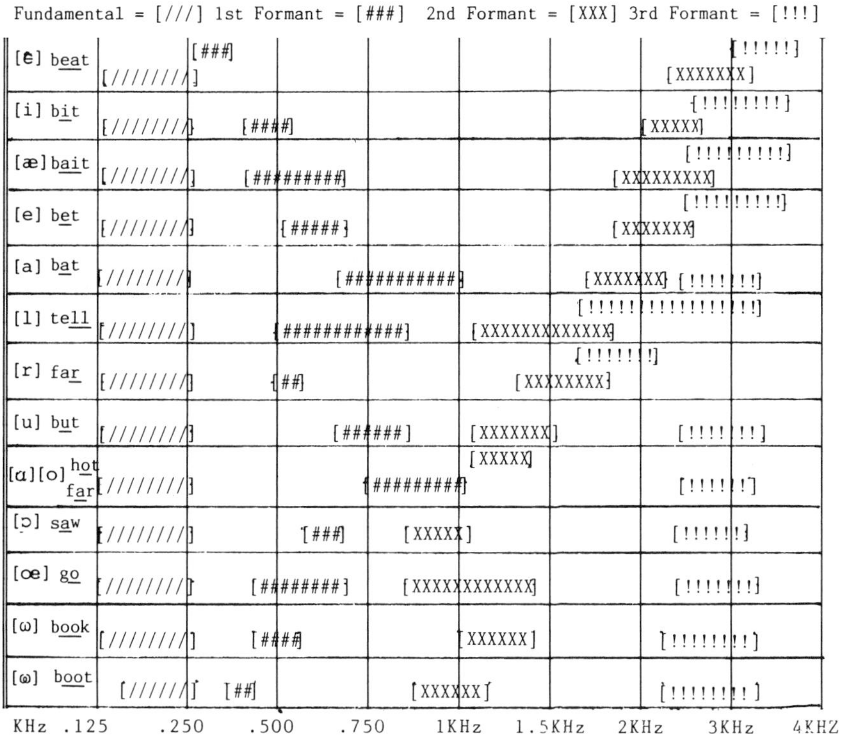

Fundamental = [///]   1st Formant = [###]   2nd Formant = [XXX]   3rd Formant = [!!!]

	.125	.250	.500	.750	1KHz	1.5KHz	2KHz	3KHz	4KHz
[e] beat	[////////]	[###]					[XXXXXXX]	[!!!!!]	
[i] bit	[////////]	[####]					[XXXXX]	{!!!!!!!!}	
[æ] bait	[////////]	[#########]				[XXXXXXXXX]		[!!!!!!!!]	
[e] bet	[////////]	{#####}				[XXXXXXX]		[!!!!!!!!]	
[a] bat	[////////]	[###########]				[XXXXXXX]	[!!!!!]		
[l] tell	[////////]	{###########}		[XXXXXXXXXXXXX]		[!!!!!!!!!!!!!]			
[r] far	[////////]	{##}		[XXXXXXXX]		{!!!!!!}			
[u] but	[////////]	[######]		[XXXXXXX]			[!!!!!]		
[a][o] hot far	[////////]	{#########}	[XXXXX]				[!!!!!]		
[ɔ] saw	[////////]	[###]	[XXXXX]				[!!!!!]		
[oe] go	[////////]	[########]	[XXXXXXXXXXX]				[!!!!!]		
[w] book	[////////]	[####]	[XXXXXX]				[!!!!!!]		
[ɯ] boot	[//////]	[##]	[XXXXXXX]				[!!!!!!]		

KHz .125   .250   .500   .750   1KHz   1.5KHz   2KHz   3KHz   4KHZ

* Data adapted from the research of Peterson and Barney [1952].

Fig. 2. Frequency Spectrum of Vowels and Semivowels.

For persons who are unable to hear above 1000 Hz the distinguishing features of the unvoiced consonants will be inaudible, although, [sh] and [ch] have low-frequency components that might permit recognition. A voiced consonant may be recognized because of low-frequency components that may be audible or because of the influence of the transition frequencies of the vowel that precedes or follows it.

The nasals, [m], [n], [ng], are voiced sounds but are emitted through the nasal passage rather than through the mouth (oral cavity). They are about as difficult to recognize as are the voiced consonants. The semivowels, [r], [l], [w], [y], all function as glides but [r] and [l] also serve the function of vowels. Example: The [r] in "river" [rivr] serves as a glide in [ri] and as a vowel in [vr], while [w] and [y] function only as glides as in "we" [wɛ] and in "you" [yω]. Because the [w] starts its glide as [ω] and proceeds to [ɛ] it has, for an instant, the acoustic characteristics of [ω]. Similarly, as [y] glides from [ɛ] to [ω] it, briefly, has the acoustic properties of [ɛ].

For most hearing impaired persons low-frequency phonemes are more easily identified than are those that require audibility in the higher frequencies. In general, this means that in terms of recognition, the phonemes rank from the easiest to the most difficult in this order: back vowels, front vowels, nasals, voiced consonants, unvoiced consonants. This also means that the acoustic energy of speech is greatest in the lower frequencies and gradually decreases for the higher frequency components of the speech signal which are the critical frequencies for phoneme recognition. The relatively weak intensity of the higher frequency components of speech, coupled with the fact that hearing-impaired persons usually have the greatest loss in the higher frequencies, makes selective amplification of these frequencies vital for the perception of speech. Robert West (1937) was acutely aware of this fact when he stated in his text book *The Rehabilitation of Speech* the following:

> "In high-frequency deafness a wave filter or tone control may be used to damp out the tones of lower frequencies. This allows the pupil-patient to give attention to the high-frequency sounds, which would otherwise be completely masked by the louder lower-frequency sounds."

In 1937 Arthur M. Wengel, an electronic research engineer with the Ray O Vac Co., Madison, Wisconsin, built a portable hearing aid, credited as being the first portable hearing aid built in the United States. (Berger 1970). As one of West's students in the late 1930's I was present when West demonstrated the use of Wengel's hearing aid on a child who, as I recall, was about 6 years old. Unaided and aided soundfield measurements were performed which showed how the frequencies most important for the child to hear had been selectively amplified so that he could learn to perceive speech and learn to produce intelligible speech.

SELECTIVE AMPLIFICATION

With pure-tone and speech audiometry the hearing needs of the client are discovered and an appropriate hearing aid is chosen based upon data provided by the manufacturer or from a hearing aid analyzer. Sound-field unaided and aided (with custom ear mold) measurements will show whether or not the gain and frequency response characteristics of the aid being considered brings the phonemes, essential for speech perception, into the audible range of the client. Figure 3 shows a typical loss and the amplification characteristics of a hearing aid in relation to the speech spectrum.

The hearing aid which provides the greatest audibility in the area most important for speech perception should be chosen. That will be the

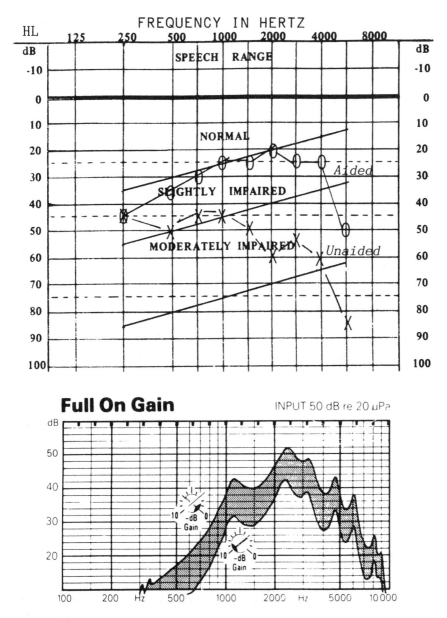

Fig. 3. TOP — Unaided and BTE aided soundfield curves. Gain of aid set at MCL, approximately at the reference test gain level of the aid. BOTTOM — Mfg's full on gain and reference test gain curves for aid used. Frequency-gain curve for the specific aid used is similar to the reference test gain curve shown above, except that it showed more gain at 4000 Hz than does the above curve.

aid with the appropriate frequency/response characteristics, sufficient gain, the proper output, and the least distortion. Will the amplification the aid provides be "transparent"? Which means, will the client hear with the aid like he did without it, only hear sounds louder? Certainly not, if greater speech intelligibility is to be achieved. The misguided practice of selecting a particular hearing aid, for a first time user, because it is the one that sounds most "natural" (read, "transparent") to him was addressed by West (1947) as follows:

> ". . . one cannot rely with confidence upon the testimony of the patient . . .
> he is inclined to compare the speech sounds that the audicle affords with
> his own distorted notion of how speech should sound rather than with the
> normal sounds of speech. He cannot be trusted to select his own aid . . ."

Returning to Figure 3, you will note that the aided frequency-gain curve rises by 15 dB from 500 Hz to 2000 Hz. This rise is consistent with the rise of the speech spectrum curve, except for a slight drop at 3000 Hz and 4000 Hz. Since we are using the standard audiogram form, that means that the higher-frequency sounds of speech are weaker than the lower-frequency sounds of speech and thus appear closer to the top of the audiogram. The Peterson and Barney data (1952) shows that for vowels, the intensity of the higher frequency second formants range from 7 to 20 dB weaker than the lower frequency first formants.

I have found that in my own speech the unvoiced consonants, except [s], [sh], and [ch], are from 12 dB to 15 dB weaker in intensity than are the vowel [ɔ] as in "*saw*", with [s] and [ch] 10 dB weaker and [sh] only 5 dB weaker than [ɔ]. These sound pressure measurements were made on the C scale of a sound level meter. From all of the evidence it seems reasonable to strive to provide amplification that gradually increases in intensity by 15 dB over the range from 500 Hz to 4000 Hz as shown by aided *real-ear* warble-tone soundfield measurements. (See Figure 3)

PHONEME RECOGNITION TESTING

When the hearing aid to be evaluated has been adjusted to the most comfortable loudness level (MCL), phoneme recognition ability may be tested. For the client with only a slight to moderate hearing-impairment, particularly in the high frequencies, the Phoneme Recognition Quick Test (See Tables 3-6) may be all that is needed to determine phoneme recognition capability. The Phoneme Recognition Quick Test presents the unvoiced consonants both when they precede and when they follow the vowel in the word. All of the vowels and unvoiced consonants are represented within the 22 words of the test. A correct response indicates that either the consonant was heard or that frequen-

Table 3
Phoneme Recognition Quick Test
List Number One - Randomizations 1-2

List I-1					List I-2				
1. patch	[p	a	ch]	= ____	1. choke	[ch	œ	k]	= ____
2. face	[f	æ	s]	= ____	2. pep	[p	e	p]	= ____
3. choke	[ch	œ	k]	= ____	3. fuss	[f	u	s]	= ____
4. kiss	[k	i	s]	= ____	4. safe	[s	æ	f]	= ____
5. thought	[th	ɔ	t]	= ____	5. feet	[f	ɛ	t]	= ____
6. pep	[p	e	p]	= ____	6. thick	[th	i	k]	= ____
7. shoot	[sh	ω	t]	= ____	7. push	[p	ω	sh]	= ____
8. caught	[c	ɔ	t]	= ____	8. face	[f	æ	s]	= ____
9. set	[s	e	t]	= ____	9. tooth	[t	ω	th]	= ____
10. tooth	[t	ω	th]	= ____	10. soak	[s	œ	k]	= ____
11. top	[t	o	p]	= ____	11. cuff	[c	u	f]	= ____
12. feet	[f	e	t]	= ____	12. top	[t	o	p]	= ____
13. took	[t	ω	k]	= ____	13. set	[s	e	t]	= ____
14. cuff	[c	u	f]	= ____	14. chop	[ch	o	p]	= ____
15. safe	[s	æ	f]	= ____	15. patch	[p	a	ch]	= ____
16. path	[p	a	th]	= ____	16. kiss	[k	i	s]	= ____
17. fuss	[f	u	s]	= ____	17. shoot	[sh	ω	t]	= ____
18. thick	[th	i	k]	= ____	18. thought	[th	ɔ	t]	= ____
19. heap	[h	e	p]	= ____	19. took	[t	ω	k]	= ____
20. chop	[ch	o	p]	= ____	20. path	[p	a	th]	= ____
21. push	[p	ω	sh]	= ____	21. heap	[h	e	p]	= ____
22. soak	[s	œ	k]	= ____	22. caught	[c	ɔ	t]	= ____

Correct responses x 1.5 = score
Auditory score = _____
Auditory—visual score = _____
Phones: _____ Soundfield: _____
(Highest score = 99%)
NAME: _____
TESTED BY: _____ DATE: _____

NOTE: These lists are made up only of vowels and unvoiced consonants. All unvoiced consonants appear at least once in both the initial position and (except for [h]) in the final position in the words.

Lists compiled by John K. Duffy (1987)

Table 4
Phoneme Recognition Quick Test
List Number One - Randomizations 3-4

List I-3

1.	thought	[th	ɔ	t]	= ____
2.	tooth	[t	ω	th]	= ____
3.	safe	[s	æ	f]	= ____
4.	chop	[ch	o	p]	= ____
5.	kiss	[k	i	s]	= ____
6.	set	[s	e	t]	= ____
7.	cuff	[c	u	f]	= ____
8.	choke	[ch	œ	k]	= ____
9.	heap	[h	e	p]	= ____
10.	face	[f	a	s]	= ____
11.	shoot	[sh	ω	t]	= ____
12.	caught	[c	ɔ	t]	= ____
13.	took	[t	ω	k]	= ____
14.	thick	[th	i	k]	= ____
15.	patch	[p	a	ch]	= ____
16.	pep	[p	e	p]	= ____
17.	top	[t	o	p]	= ____
18.	path	[p	a	th]	= ____
19.	push	[p	ω	sh]	= ____
20.	feet	[f	ɛ	t]	= ____
21.	fuss	[f	u	s]	= ____
22.	soak	[s	œ	k]	= ____

List I-4

1.	feet	[f	ɛ	t]	= ____
2.	push	[p	ω	sh]	= ____
3.	soak	[s	œ	k]	= ____
4.	set	[s	e	t]	= ____
5.	took	[t	ω	k]	= ____
6.	kiss	[k	i	s]	= ____
7.	caught	[c	ɔ	t]	= ____
8.	pep	[p	e	p]	= ____
9.	safe	[s	æ	f]	= ____
10.	top	[t	o	p]	= ____
11.	face	[f	æ	s]	= ____
12.	chop	[ch	o	p]	= ____
13.	shoot	[sh	ω	t]	= ____
14.	path	[p	a	th]	= ____
15.	choke	[ch	œ	k]	= ____
16.	fuss	[f	u	s]	= ____
17.	thick	[th	i	k]	= ____
18.	tooth	[t	ω	th]	= ____
19.	cuff	[c	u	f]	= ____
20.	patch	[p	a	ch]	= ____
22.	thought	[th	ɔ	t]	= ____
22.	heap	[h	ɛ	p]	= ____

Correct responses x 1.5 = score
Auditory score: I-3 = _____ I-4 = _____
Auditory—visual score: I-3 _____ I-4 _____
Phones: _____ Soundfield: _____
(Highest score = 99%)
NAME: _____
TESTED BY: _____ DATE: _____

NOTE: These lists are made up only of vowels and unvoiced consonants. All unvoiced consonants appear at least once in both the initial position and (except for [h]) in the final position in the words.

Lists compiled by John K. Duffy (1987)

Table 5
Phoneme Recognition Quick Test
List Number Two - Randomization 1-2

List II-1

1.	teeth	[t	ε	th	]	= ____
2.	pace	[p	æ	s	]	= ____
3.	thatch	[th	a	ch	]	= ____
4.	fish	[f	i	sh	]	= ____
5.	tough	[t	u	f	]	= ____
6.	fetch	[f	e	ch	]	= ____
7.	hut	[h	u	t	]	= ____
8.	chap	[ch	a	p	]	= ____
9.	shape	[sh	æ	p	]	= ____
10.	cheek	[ch	ε	k	]	= ____
11.	shed	[sh	e	d	]	= ____
12.	sick	[s	i	k	]	= ____
13.	pot	[p	o	t	]	= ____
14.	foot	[f	ω	t	]	= ____
15.	soap	[s	œ	p	]	= ____
16.	cop	[c	o	p	]	= ____
17.	joke	[j	œ	k	]	= ____
18.	sauce	[s	ɔ	s	]	= ____
19.	toot	[t	ω	t	]	= ____
20.	cough	[c	ɔ	f	]	= ____
21.	couth	[c	ω	th	]	= ____
22.	sought	[s	ɔ	t	]	= ____

List II-2

1.	tough	[t	u	f	]	= ____
2.	chap	[ch	a	p	]	= ____
3.	sick	[s	i	k	]	= ____
4.	cop	[c	o	p	]	= ____
5.	thatch	[th	a	ch	]	= ____
6.	cough	[c	ɔ	f	]	= ____
7.	pace	[p	æ	s	]	= ____
8.	couth	[c	ω	th	]	= ____
9.	cheek	[ch	ε	k	]	= ____
10.	foot	[f	ω	t	]	= ____
11.	fish	[f	i	sh	]	= ____
12.	hut	[h	u	t	]	= ____
13.	shape	[sh	æ	p	]	= ____
14.	sought	[s	ɔ	t	]	= ____
15.	pot	[p	o	t	]	= ____
16.	shed	[sh	e	d	]	= ____
17.	teeth	[t	ε	th	]	= ____
18.	fetch	[f	ε	ch	]	= ____
19.	soap	[s	œ	p	]	= ____
20.	toot	[t	ω	t	]	= ____
21.	poke	[p	œ	k	]	= ____
22.	sauce	[s	ɔ	s	]	= ____

Correct responses x 1.5 = score
Auditory score: II-1 = _____ II-2 = _____
Auditory—visual score: II-1 _____ II-2 _____
Phones: _____ Soundfield: _____
(Highest score = 99%)
NAME: _____
TESTED BY: _____ DATE: _____

NOTE: These lists are made up only of vowels and unvoiced consonants. All unvoiced consonants appear at least once in both the initial position and (except for [h]) in the final position in the words.

Lists compiled by John K. Duffy (1987)

Table 6
Phoneme Recognition Quick Test
List Number Two - Randomizations 3-4

List II-3

#	Word	Phonemes	=
1.	sauce	[s ɔ s]	= ___
2.	fetch	[f e ch]	= ___
3.	teeth	[t ε th]	= ___
4.	poke	[p œ k]	= ___
5.	sought	[s ɔ t]	= ___
6.	fish	[f i sh]	= ___
7.	tough	[t u f]	= ___
8.	cop	[c o p]	= ___
9.	couth	[c ω th]	= ___
10.	foot	[f ω t]	= ___
11.	shape	[sh æ p]	= ___
12.	pot	[p o t]	= ___
13.	soap	[s œ p]	= ___
14.	sick	[s i k]	= ___
15.	chap	[ch a p]	= ___
16.	toot	[t ω t]	= ___
17.	thatch	[th a ch]	= ___
18.	shed	[sh e d]	= ___
19.	hut	[h u t]	= ___
20.	cheek	[ch ε k]	= ___
21.	pace	[p æ s]	= ___
22.	cough	[c ɔ f]	= ___

List II-4

#	Word	Phonemes	=
1.	fish	[f i sh]	= ___
2.	sought	[s ɔ t]	= ___
3.	chap	[ch a p]	= ___
4.	sauce	[s ɔ s]	= ___
5.	foot	[f ω t]	= ___
6.	poke	[p œ k]	= ___
7.	shape	[sh æ p]	= ___
8.	thatch	[th a ch]	= ___
9.	cough	[c ɔ f]	= ___
10.	cheek	[ch ε k]	= ___
11.	shed	[sh e d]	= ___
12.	couth	[c ω th]	= ___
13.	pot	[p o t]	= ___
14.	teeth	[t ε th]	= ___
15.	pace	[p æ s]	= ___
16.	hut	[h u t]	= ___
17.	toot	[t ω t]	= ___
18.	soap	[s œ p]	= ___
19.	cop	[c o p]	= ___
20.	tough	[t u f]	= ___
21.	fetch	[f e ch]	= ___
22.	sick	[s i k]	= ___

Correct responses x 1.5 = score
Auditory score: II-3 = _____ II-4 = _____
Auditory—visual score: II-3 _____ II-4 _____
Phones: _____ Soundfield: _____
(Highest score = 99%)
NAME: _____
TESTED BY: _____ DATE: _____

NOTE: These lists are made up only of vowels and unvoiced consonants. All unvoiced consonants appear at least once in both the initial position and (except for [h]) in the final position in the words.

Lists compiled by John K. Duffy (1987)

cies were heard that were produced as the consonant approached or receded from the vowel. These frequencies are called "transition frequencies (influences)". When these sounds are audible they often enable the client to perceive the word or a portion of the word.

By noting the client's correct responses, ommissions or substitutions, a record can be kept for guidance in carrying out auditory and auditory visual training and in computing the client's speech perception index. (To be discussed later).

The two lists of the Phoneme Recognition Inventory (See Tables 7-10) were designed for the client with a moderate and severe hearing impairment. Each list contains 33 words. All of the phonemes of English speech appear in various vowel consonant relationships. These lists provide a generous sample of the speech sound combinations found in everyday speech and provide a strong indication of the client's phoneme recognition ability.

The Phoneme Recognition Inventory and the Quick Test can be administered with live voice, audio tapes or video tapes. (Speech & Hearing Habilitation Films, Inc.) A carrier phrase preceding each word is not recommended for these tests. The conventional practice of repeating the phrase "Say the word" or "You will say" before each word is unnecessary, time consuming, and tiresome for the testor and boring for the testee. (Martin et al., 1962).

In administering the tests, present each word at about the same intensity level with sufficient time between presentations for the client to respond. Have the client repeat the words that he thinks he hears. Under some circumstances having the client both speak and write the test words may be advisable. Audio tape recording of the client's responses is recommended. This allows for the scoring and analysis of the client's phoneme recognition test responses as well as for comparing auditory with auditory-visual responses. Although it is common knowledge that hearing-impaired listeners usually have greater speech perception ability when they are watching a speaker than otherwise, the auditory-visual measurements of speech perception ability have, in general, been ignored by the hearing care practioner. We believe that both auditory and auditory-visual measurements should be made as standard procedure for all clients, except for those who get very high auditory scores.

For the practioner who is actively engaged in hearing rehabilitation the Phoneme Recognition tests are a very useful tool. The record of the client's response to each word will show the phonemes and sound combinations that were recognized through audition alone as well as the phonemes that were recognized when auditory cues were accompanied by visual cues through lip reading. With this information, auditory and auditory-visual training designed to improve speech perception can proceed.

Table 7
Phoneme Recgonition Inventory/List Number One - Randomizations 1-2

List I-1

1. feel — [f ɛ l]   = _____
2. map — [m a p]   = _____
3. waifs — [w æ fs]   = _____
4. might — [m ai t]   = _____
5. that — [th a t]   = _____
6. stops — [st o ps]   = _____
7. fads — [f a dz]   = _____
8. which — [wh i ch]   = _____
9. vision — [v i zh u n]   = _____
10. pouch — [p oω ch]   = _____
11. chess — [ch e s]   = _____
12. rock — [r o k]   = _____
13. thin — [th i n]   = _____
14. shoot — [sh ω t]   = _____
15. bird — [b r d]   = _____
16. skip — [sk i p]   = _____
17. speck — [sp e k]   = _____
18. vast — [v a st]   = _____
19. gave — [g æ v]   = _____
20. leash — [l ɛ sh]   = _____
21. dig — [d i g]   = _____
22. bathes — [b æ th z]   = _____
23. took — [t ω k]   = _____
24. heats — [h ɛ ts]   = _____
25. lathe — [l æ th]   = _____
26. speak — [sp ɛ k]   = _____
27. tub — [t u b]   = _____
28. yes — [y e s]   = _____
29. sing — [s i ng]   = _____
30. call — [c ɔ l]   = _____
31. faiths — [f æ ths]   = _____
32. folks — [f œ ks]   = _____
33. joy — [j ɔi]   = _____

List I-2

1. that — [th a t]   = _____
2. chess — [ch e s]   = _____
3. skip — [sk i p]   = _____
4. dig — [d i g]   = _____
5. speak — [sp ɛ k]   = _____
6. faiths — [f æ ths]   = _____
7. waifs — [w æ fs]   = _____
8. shoot — [sh ω t]   = _____
9. which — [wh i ch]   = _____
10. gave — [g æ v]   = _____
11. heats — [h ɛ ts]   = _____
12. sing — [s i ng]   = _____
13. feel — [f ɛ l]   = _____
14. stops — [st o ps]   = _____
15. rock — [r o k]   = _____
16. speck — [sp e k]   = _____
17. bathes — [b æ thz]   = _____
18. tub — [t u b]   = _____
19. folks — [f œ ks]   = _____
20. might — [m ai t]   = _____
21. vision — [v i zh u n]   = _____
22. bird — [b r d]   = _____
22. leash — [l ɛ sh]   = _____
24. lathe — [l æ th]   = _____
25. call — [c ɔ l]   = _____
26. map — [m a p]   = _____
27. fads — [f a dz]   = _____
28. thin — [th i n]   = _____
29. vast — [v a st]   = _____
30. took — [t ω k]   = _____
31. yes — [y e s]   = _____
32. joy — [j ɔi]   = _____
33. pouch — [p oω ch]   = _____

Auditory score: I-1 = _____ I-2 = _____
Auditory—visual score: I-1 _____ I-2 _____
Phones: _____ Soundfield: _____
NAME: _____
TESTED BY: _____ DATE: _____

NOTE: These lists include all English sounds with consonants appearing in the initial and final position in words. Give one point for each phoneme, diphthong and consonant blend. Each part of blend = ½ point. Highest score 100%.

Table 8
Phoneme Recognition Inventory/List Number One - Randomizations 3-4

List I-3

#	word	transcription	=	score
1.	stops	[st o ps]	=	_____
2.	bird	[b r d]	=	_____
3.	chess	[ch e s]	=	_____
4.	gave	[g æ v]	=	_____
5.	took	[t ω k]	=	_____
6.	tub	[t u b]	=	_____
7.	faiths	[f æ ths]	=	_____
8.	map	[m a p]	=	_____
9.	that	[th a t]	=	_____
10.	speak	[sp ε k]	=	_____
11.	which	[wh i ch]	=	_____
12.	rock	[r o k]	=	_____
13.	pouch	[p oω ch]	=	_____
14.	dig	[d i g]	=	_____
15.	heats	[h ε ts]	=	_____
16.	yes	[y e s]	=	_____
17.	folks	[f œ ks]	=	_____
18.	feel	[f ε l]	=	_____
19.	waifs	[w æ fs]	=	_____
20.	fads	[f a dz]	=	_____
21.	call	[c ɔ l]	=	_____
22.	vision	[v i zh u n]	=	_____
23.	thin	[th i n]	=	_____
24.	skip	[sk i p]	=	_____
25.	vast	[v a st]	=	_____
26.	bathes	[b æ th z]	=	_____
27.	lathe	[l æ th]	=	_____
28.	sing	[s i ng]	=	_____
29.	joy	[j ɔi]	=	_____
30.	might	[m ai t]	=	_____
31.	shoot	[sh ω t]	=	_____
32.	speck	[sp e k]	=	_____
33.	leash	[l ε sh]	=	_____

List I-4

#	word	transcription	=	score
1.	feel	[f ε l]	=	_____
2.	waifs	[w æ fs]	=	_____
1.	that	[th a t]	=	_____
4.	fads	[f a ds]	=	_____
5.	vision	[v i zh u n]	=	_____
6.	rock	[r o k]	=	_____
7.	shoot	[sh ω t]	=	_____
8.	skip	[sk i p]	=	_____
9.	vast	[v a st]	=	_____
10.	leash	[l ε sh]	=	_____
11.	bathes	[b æ thz]	=	_____
12.	heats	[h ε ts]	=	_____
13.	yes	[y e s]	=	_____
14.	call	[c ɔ l]	=	_____
15.	speak	[sp ε k]	=	_____
16.	folks	[f œ ks]	=	_____
17.	joy	[j ɔi]	=	_____
18.	map	[m a p]	=	_____
19.	might	[m ai t]	=	_____
20.	stops	[st o ps]	=	_____
21.	which	[wh i ch]	=	_____
22.	chess	[ch e s]	=	_____
23.	pouch	[p oω ch]	=	_____
24.	thin	[th i n]	=	_____
25.	bird	[b r d]	=	_____
26.	speck	[sp e k]	=	_____
27.	gave	[g æ v]	=	_____
28.	dig	[d i g]	=	_____
29.	took	[t ωι k]	=	_____
30.	lathe	[l æ th]	=	_____
31.	tub	[t u b]	=	_____
32.	sing	[s i ng]	=	_____
32.	faiths	[f æ ths]	=	_____

Auditory score: I-3 = _____ I-4 = _____
Auditory—visual score: I-3 _____ I-4 _____
Phones: _____ Soundfield: _____
NAME: _____
TESTED BY: _____ DATE: _____

NOTE: These lists include all English sounds with consonants appearing in the initial and final position in words. Give one point for each phoneme, diphthong and consonant blend. Each part of blend = ½ point. Highest score 100%.

Table 9
Phoneme Recognition Inventory/List Number Two - Randomizations 1-2

List II-1						List II-2					
1.	leaf	[l	ε	f]	= _____	1.	than	[t̶h̶	a	n]	= _____
2.	keeps	[k̄	ε̄	p̄s̄]	= _____	2.	face	[f̄	ǣ	s̄]	= _____
3.	vague	[v̄	ǣ	ḡ]	= _____	1.	time	[t̄	āi	m̄]	= _____
4.	such	[s̄	ū	c̄h̄]	= _____	4.	gnat	[n̄	ā	t̄]	= _____
5.	than	[t̶h̶	ā	n̄]	= _____	5.	spots	[s̄p̄	ō	t̄s̄]	= _____
6.	but	[b̄	ū	t̄]	= _____	6.	wasps	[w̄	ā	s̄p̄s̄]	= _____
7.	sheet	[s̄h̄	ε̄	t̄]	= _____	7.	chip	[c̄h̄	ī	p̄]	= _____
8.	tsar	[z̄	ā	r̄]	= _____	8.	leisure	[l̄	ε̄	z̄h̄ r]	= _____
9.	face	[f̄	ǣ	s̄]	= _____	9.	such	[s̄	ū	c̄h̄]	= _____
10.	when	[w̄h̄	ē	n̄]	= _____	10.	tsar	[z̄	ā	r̄]	= _____
11.	give	[ḡ	ī	v̄]	= _____	11.	thick	[t̄h̄	ī	k̄]	= _____
12.	thick	[t̄h̄	ī	k̄]	= _____	12.	tooth	[t̄	ω̄	t̄h̄]	= _____
13.	time	[t̄	āi	m̄]	= _____	13.	dirt	[d̄	r	t̄]	= _____
14.	wrong	[r̄	ɔ̄	n̄ḡ]	= _____	14.	picks	[p̄	ī	k̄s̄]	= _____
15.	babe	[b̄	ǣ	b̄]	= _____	15.	yachts	[ȳ	a	t̄s̄]	= _____
16.	tooth	[t̄	ω̄	t̄h̄]	= _____	16.	vague	[v̄	ǣ	ḡ]	= _____
17.	gnat	[n̄	ā	t̄]	= _____	17.	sheet	[s̄h̄	ε̄	t̄]	= _____
18.	loss	[l̄	ɔ̄	t̄s̄]	= _____	18.	give	[ḡ	ī	v̄]	= _____
19.	could	[c̄	ω̄	d̄]	= _____	19.	babe	[b̄	ǣ	b̄]	= _____
20.	dirt	[d̄	r	t̄]	= _____	20.	could	[c̄	ω̄	d̄]	= _____
21.	spots	[s̄p̄	ō	t̄s̄]	= _____	21.	steep	[s̄t̄	ε̄	p̄]	= _____
22.	hatch	[h̄	ā	c̄h̄]	= _____	22.	jail	[j̄	ǣ	l̄]	= _____
23.	steep	[s̄t̄	ε̄	p̄]	= _____	23.	chowder	[c̄h̄	ōω	d̄r̄]	= _____
24.	picks	[p̄	ī	k̄s̄]	= _____	24.	keeps	[k̄	ε̄	p̄s̄]	= _____
25.	wasps	[w̄	ā	s̄p̄s̄]	= _____	25.	but	[b̄	ū	t̄]	= _____
26.	scope	[s̄c̄	œ̄	p̄]	= _____	26.	when	[w̄h̄	ē	n̄]	= _____
27.	jail	[j̄	ǣ	l̄]	= _____	27.	wrong	[r̄	ɔ̄	n̄ḡ]	= _____
28.	kept	[k̄	ē	p̄t̄]	= _____	28.	loss	[l̄	ɔ̄	s̄]	= _____
29.	chip	[c̄h̄	ī	p̄]	= _____	29.	hatch	[h̄	ā	c̄h̄]	= _____
30.	toil	[t̄	ɔ̄i	l̄]	= _____	30.	scope	[s̄c̄	œ̄	p̄]	= _____
31.	chowder	[c̄h̄	ōω	d̄r̄]	= _____	31.	toil	[t̄	ɔ̄i	l̄]	= _____
32.	yachts	[ȳ	a	t̄s̄]	= _____	32.	leaf	[l̄	ε̄	f̄]	= _____
33.	leisure	[l̄	ε̄	z̄h̄ r]	= _____	32.	kept	[k̄	ē	p̄t̄]	= _____
		_	_	_ _	= _____			_	_	_	= _____

Auditory score: II-1 = _____ II-2 = _____
Auditory—visual score: II-1 _____ II-2 _____
Phones: _____ Soundfield: _____
NAME: _____
TESTED BY: _____ DATE: _____

NOTE: These lists include all English sounds with consonants appearing in the initial and final position in words. Give one point for each phoneme, diphthong and consonant blend. Each part of blend = ½ point. Highest score 100%.

Table 10
Phoneme Recognition Inventory/List Number Two - Randomizations 3-4

List II-3						List II-4				
1.	gnat	[n	a	t]	= _____	2.	time	[t	ɑi	m]	= _____
2.	tsar	[z̄	ā	r̄]	= _____	2.	such	[s̄	ū	ch]	= _____
3.	chip	[c̄h	ī	p̄]	= _____	3.	spots	[s̄p	ō	t̄s]	= _____
4.	dirt	[d̄	r̄	t̄]	= _____	4.	thick	[t̄h	ī	k̄]	= _____
5.	vague	[v̄	ǣ	ḡ]	= _____	5.	yachts	[ȳ	a	t̄s]	= _____
6.	kept	[k̄	e	p̄t]	= _____	6.	steep	[s̄t	ε̄	p̄]	= _____
7.	picks	[p̄	ī	k̄s]	= _____	7.	wrong	[r̄	ɔ	ng]	= _____
8.	but	[b̄	ū	t]	= _____	8.	face	[f̄	ǣ	s̄]	= _____
9.	loss	[l̄	ɔ̄	s̄]	= _____	9.	chip	[c̄h	ī	p̄]	= _____
10.	toil	[t̄	ī	l̄]	= _____	10.	tsar	[z̄	ā	r̄]	= _____
11.	than	[t̶h̶	ā	n̄]	= _____	11.	vague	[v̄	ǣ	ḡ]	= _____
12.	jail	[j̄	ǣ	l̄]	= _____	12.	sheet	[s̄h	ε̄	t̄]	= _____
13.	time	[t̄	ɑi	m̄]	= _____	13.	chowder	[c̄h	ōω	d̄r]	= _____
14.	wasps	[w̄	a	sps]	= _____	14.	give	[ḡ	ī	v̄]	= _____
15.	babe	[b̄	ǣ	b̄]	= _____	15.	kept	[k̄	e	p̄t]	= _____
16.	such	[s̄	ū	ch]	= _____	16.	babe	[b̄	ǣ	b̄]	= _____
17.	tooth	[t̄	ω	th]	= _____	17.	leaf	[l̄	ε̄	f̄]	= _____
18.	yachts	[ȳ	a	t̄s]	= _____	18.	than	[t̶h̶	a	n̄]	= _____
19.	give	[ḡ	ī	v̄]	= _____	19.	wasps	[w̄	a	sps]	= _____
20.	steep	[s̄t	ε̄	p̄]	= _____	20.	tooth	[t̄	ω	th]	= _____
21.	when	[wh	e	n̄]	= _____	21.	could	[c̄	ω	d̄]	= _____
22.	hatch	[h̄	a	ch]	= _____	22.	jail	[j̄	ǣ	l̄]	= _____
23.	chowder	[c̄h	ōω	d̄r]	= _____	23.	keeps	[k̄	ε̄	ps]	= _____
24.	wrong	[r̄	ɔ̄	ng]	= _____	24.	scope	[s̄c	œ̄	p̄]	= _____
25.	scope	[s̄c	œ̄	p̄]	= _____	25.	gnat	[n̄	a	t]	= _____
26.	leaf	[l̄	ε̄	f̄]	= _____	26.	toil	[t̄	ɔ̄i	l̄]	= _____
27.	face	[f̄	ǣ	s̄]	= _____	27.	leisure	[l̄	ε̄	zh r]	= _____
28.	spots	[s̄p	ō	t̄s]	= _____	28.	dirt	[d̄	r̄	t̄]	= _____
29.	leisure	[l̄	ε̄	zh r]	= _____	29.	but	[b̄	ū	t]	= _____
30.	thick	[t̄h	ī	k̄]	= _____	30.	loss	[l̄	ɔ̄	s̄]	= _____
31.	sheet	[s̄h	ε̄	t̄]	= _____	31.	picks	[p̄	ī	k̄s]	= _____
32.	could	[c̄	ω	d̄]	= _____	32.	hatch	[h̄	a	ch]	= _____
33.	keeps	[k̄	ε̄	ps]	= _____	33.	when	[wh	e	n̄]	= _____
		___	___	___	= _____			___	___	___	= _____

Auditory score: II-3 = _____ II-4 = _____
Auditory—visual score: II-3 _____ II-4 _____
Phones: _____ Soundfield: _____
NAME: _____
TESTED BY: _____ DATE: _____

NOTE: These lists include all English sounds with consonants appearing in the initial and final position in words. Give one point for each phoneme, diphthong and consonant blend. Each part of blend = 1/2 point. Highest score = 100%.

PURE-TONE SOUNDFIELD AUDIOMETRY

For many years after West (1947) proposed, in the 1930's, the use of pure-tone soundfield audiometry for hearing aid evaluations, those who opposed the procedure claimed that standing waves and head movements of the subject made such measurements unreliable. Experience has shown that their fears were unfounded. Pure-tone soundfield audiometry, performed in a sound absorbent room using warbled or automatically pulsed tones, is now a generally accepted procedure for measuring the amplification provided by a hearing aid.

In conducting soundfield measurements the loud-speaker should be located in a corner of the sound room at about the ear level of the client who will be placed facing the loud-speaker at a distance of one meter. The client's head must be held in the same position during the testing. A head rest or ''jig'' attached to the chair for the purpose of holding the head in place, is recommended.

Unaided and aided audiometric measurements, using tonal signals and speech signals, are conducted as in headphone audiometry. A properly calibrated soundfield system may yield similar, but not necessarily the same, threshold measurements as found for the composite better ear of the client as measured through headphones. Because the differences in threshold intensity levels between unaided and aided responses is what is being measured, a difference, if any, between the unaided better ear measurements in a soundfield and those obtained with headphones, is not relevant when comparing aided soundfield responses with unaided soundfield threshold measurements.

However, headphone threshold measurements do play a role when the aid is worn in the poorer ear. The unaided soundfield threshold responses represent the better ear while the aided threshold responses represent the aided poorer ear. The difference between these two threshold measurements plus the difference between the poorer and better ear headphone threshold measurements represent the gain of the aid (see Figure 4).

Another method is to conduct the unaided soundfield test of the poorer ear while a headphone is used to apply narrow band masking to the better ear. The poorer ear remains unoccluded for the soundfield measurements. This use of masking enables one to obtain an accurate threshold for the unaided poorer ear. After performing the aided soundfield measurements, the two thresholds may be compared to determine the amount of gain being provided by the instrument. It is wise to use masking only during the unaided test. The use of masking during the aided test may reduce the measured gain of the aid due to the central masking phenomenon.

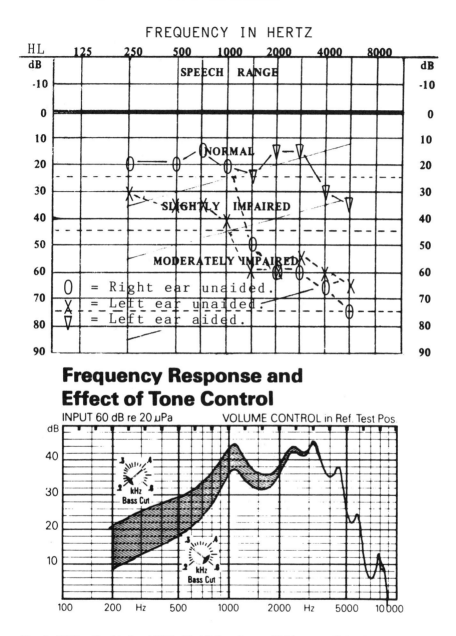

Fig. 4. TOP — Unaided and BTE aided (left ear) soundfield curves. Gain of aid set at MCL, approximately at the reference test gain level of aid. The composite better ear unaided soundfield curve represents right ear below 2000 Hz and left ear above 2000 Hz. The aided curve represents the left ear aided response above 1000 Hz. The frequencies below 1000 Hz are heard normally in unaided right ear. The frequencies above 1000 Hz are heard in aided left ear. The user is very pleased with the aid. (Full base cut used, see lower curve).

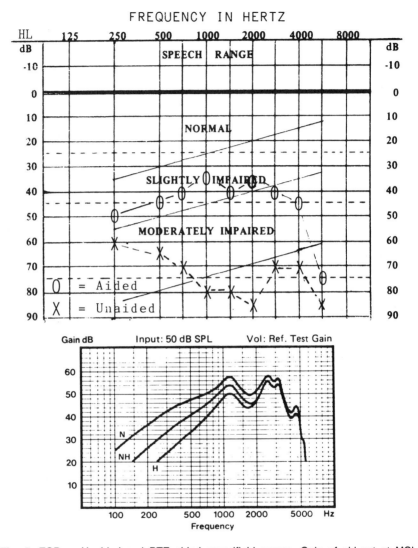

Fig. 5. TOP — Unaided and BTE aided soundfield curves. Gain of aid set at MCL, approximately at the reference test gain level of aid. BOTTOM — Mfg's response curve for aid used at NH setting. User has a congenital sensorineural hearing impairment with usable hearing only in left ear. Test data follows:

Unaided SRT = 75 dB   Aided SRT = 35 dB

Aided Phoneme Recognition Inventory scores:

Auditory: Phoneme scoring = 76%	Loss (PRL) = 24%
Whole word scoring = 42%	PRL = 58%
Auditory-visual: Phoneme scoring = 93%	PRL = 7%
Whole word scoring = 81%	PRL = 19%

Unaided Speech Perception Index (SPI) = 100 (Severe loss)
Aided SPI (auditory) = 60 (Moderate loss)
Aided SPI (auditory-visual) = 45 (Slight loss)

It should be kept in mind that the pattern of aided responses, with the gain of the aid at MCL, will appear at different levels on the audiogram depending upon the degree of hearing impairment (see Figures 3, 4, 5). If, with amplification, it lies in the NORMAL level, the client will hear speech at or near normal intensities. If it lies in the SLIGHTLY IMPAIRED area, a higher intensity of speech will be required for speech perception. If it lies in the MODERATELY IMPAIRED area the speaker will need to be closer to the listener or speak with greater intensity and visual cues through lip reading may be needed in order to make speech intelligible. The client in the SEVERELY IMPAIRED area will need to use all of the auditory, visual, and contextual cues available in order to understand speech.

The aided warble-tone soundfield pattern of amplification that my colleagues and I have found to be most beneficial for our clients is a most comfortable loudness level pattern that parallels, as closely as possible, the frequency response curve of the speech spectrum between 250 Hz and 4000 Hz. Because of the frequency-gain characteristics of most hearing aids, the gain of the aid often decreases above 3000 Hz or 4000 Hz (see Figure 3).

Speech audiometry, when used as the only procedure for evaluating hearing aids, has been proven to be highly unreliable. Furthermore, without tonal, or some other frequency related narrow-band signal soundfield measurements, the real-ear frequency-gain characteristics of the hearing aid being evaluated remain unknown.

We believe that warble-tone soundfield audiometry is the most realistic method for evaluating the performance of a hearing aid in relation to what is actually being heard by the person using it.

The present day use of the computer probe-tube microphone instrumentation for measuring hearing aid responses is an attempt to measure the frequency-gain characteristics of a hearing aid as influenced by the resonance of the subject's ear canal, but without discovering how the user actually hears with the aid. This system is purported to be more relevant to hearing aid fitting than data from conventional hearing analyzers or the Kemar® manikin and is considered, by some, to be a substitute for soundfield measurements. A few questions in need of answers about this device are:

1 In open ear fittings does the presence of a tube in the ear canal change ear canal resonance?

2 Does putting the probe tube through the vent of what would otherwise be a vented mold affect ear canal resonance?

3 Can the probe tube be placed alongside a tight mold in a very narrow ear canal, particularly that of a young child?

4 Can the probe tube be placed beside a tight mold without the tube being flattened or without allowing feedback squeal?

5   Is drilling a hole in the mold to permit probe tube insertion practical on a routine basis?

6   How does the insertion-gain response of the aid relate to the pattern and degree of the subject's hearing impairment?

7   How does the insertion frequency-gain readout relate to what the subject really hears?

8   How are phoneme recognition tests performed with this instrumentation?

9   How can the computer probe-tube microphone instrumentation perform a *real ear* measurement without involving the entire hearing mechanism of the subject, not just the ear canal?

10   Can computer probe-tube microphone measurements be made on a dead ear?

11   Why incur the expense of such a system when a hearing aid analyzer can provide essential hearing aid performance data and conventional audiometric instrumentation is all that is required to perform warble-tone and speech soundfield audiometry, which actually does measure the client's *real* auditory responses?

In describing various hearing aid selection approaches in Chapter I Zelnick mentioned the Harvard Report (Davis et al. 1947) and suggested that I would have more to say about it. These are my comments:

In this government supported study, Davis and his associates concluded that hearing aids with either a flat response or a response that showed a rise of 6 dB per octave would provide the best electroacoustic characteristics for all or most hearing aid users and that:

> ". . . we have disproved the fundamental assumption of the desirability of "selective amplification" based on the characteristics of the individual's audiogram."

Selective amplification was widely accepted until the Harvard Report. Hearing aid manufacturers generally ignored the report's recommendations, but many in the academic and clinical community were unfortunately mislead. As a professor of audiology at Brooklyn College of the City University of New York, I described the Harvard study to my graduate students as an example of surprisingly poor research design and execution and pointed out the misleading conclusions drawn from the study.

Besides the small number of ears used (25) and the odd assortment of types of loss and audiometric patterns, the most glaring flaws in the research were:

1 A Master Hearing Aid unlike any wearable hearing aids then available was used.

2 Earphones rather than miniature hearing aid receivers and custom earmolds were used and the frequency response characteristics of the Master Hearing Aid were not related to "real-ear" soundfield measurements.

3 Fletcher (1953) showed that the "real-ear" (orthtelephonic) response of the Master Hearing Aid used in the Harvard Study was humped with amplification at 500 Hz at an intensity 10 dB greater than at 2000 Hz, for the flat setting, while the "high pass 6 dB" curve was practically flat from 500 Hz to 2000 Hz.

4 The speech discrimination tests were performed with the Harvard PB Word Lists. The lack of reliability of such tests, using all-or-none whole word scoring, is well established (Duffy 1967).

Fortunately, technological advances in electronics, acoustics, engineering and manufacturing were not deterred by the Harvard Study and today we have hearing aids with amazing adjustability and quality. It is our responsibility to utilize these marvelous instruments to the fullest.

THE SPEECH SPECTRUM CURVE

The goal of amplification should be to make audible as many of the sounds of speech as possible which will make speech intelligible for the hearing-impaired person. Here are some factors to consider:

The second formants for the vowels and semivowels contain the most critical frequencies for identification and fall as low as 840 Hz for men and as high as 3200 Hz for children.

The third formants for the vowels and semivowels range as low as 1690 Hz for men and as high as 3730 Hz for children.

First formants for the vowels and semivowels range in intensity from 7 dB to 20 dB more than the second formants and second formants range in intensity from 4 dB to 27 dB more than third formants. This means that the intensity of amplification must increase as the frequency increases.

Considering the relative weakness of the unvoiced consonants over the voiced sounds and the weakness of the second formants over the first formants, we recommend that a gradual intensity increase of 15 dB between 500 Hz and 4000 Hz be the target pattern of amplification in order to achieve the highest level of phoneme recognition. We call this pattern the Speech Spectrum Curve. Figures 3, 4, and 5 show how this curve follows the speech spectrum guidelines for the client whose soundfield audiogram is plotted. We believe that the speech spectrum pattern of amplification is the one best suited to improve the client's phoneme recognition ability. The above recommendation comes under the heading of prescription fitting.

For the sake of comparison, Figure 6 shows four prescription fitting curves. They are: One Third Gain Rule; One Half Gain Rule; Mirror; Speech Spectrum. It can be seen in Figure 6 that the Mirror curve and the Speech Spectrum curve come closest to providing the greatest amplification in the critical area for phoneme recognition. The One Half Gain Rule curve provided more amplification below 1000 Hz than advisable and the One Third Gain Rule curve drops markedly in the critical phoneme recognition area and is clearly inadequate. No situation comes to mind where it would apply.

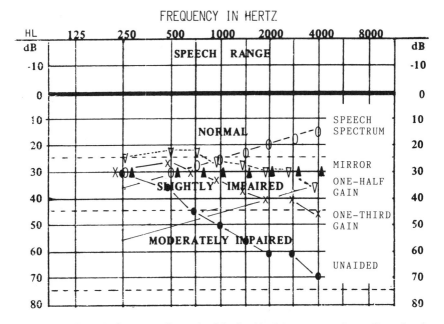

Fig. 6. The Speech Spectrum Curve (top) is the ideal frequency-gain configuration for phoneme recognition. However, in practice, the gain of most hearing aids stays the same or becomes lower for frequencies above 2000 Hz. Of course, the gain and output of the aid must be adjusted to the user's MCL and LDL. In general, frequency-gain responses which fall between the Speech Spectrum Curve and the Mirror Curve are best suited for phoneme recognition. The One-half Gain Curve provides more amplification of the frequencies below 1000 Hz than appropriate and the One-third Gain Curve is detrimental for speech perception because its lack of sufficient amplification of critical high frequency speech sounds either leaves them inaudible to the user or they are masked by the amplification of the frequencies below 1000 Hz.

A PROCEDURE FOR HEARING AID SELECTION USING SOUNDFIELD AUDIOMETRY

Equipment: audiometer; amplifier; loud-speaker(s); VCR-TV; audio tape recorder; audio tape player (see Figure 7).

After headphone audiometric tests, select the hearing aid, based upon data from the manufacturer of the aid and/or data from a hearing aid analyzer, or other source, which appears to be best suited to meet the needs of the client.

We recommend that the target for the frequency-gain response of the aid selected follow the Speech Spectrum curve (see Figures 3, 4, and 5), and for calculating the overall gain requirements of the aid, we recommend the use of the Zelnick gain formulae (see Chapter I).

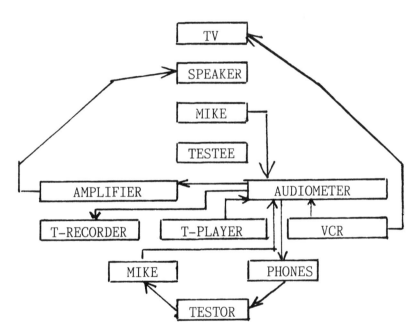

Fig. 7. Soundfield Audiometric Instrumentation.
Capabilities:
1. Warble tones and/or noise from audiometer, to amplifier, to speaker.
2. Live voice to audiometer, to amplifier, to speaker.
3. Audio taped speech signal to audiometer, to amplifier, to speaker.
4. VCR audio taped speech signal to audiometer, to amplifier, to speaker.
5. VCR video taped speech signal to TV.
6. Testee's responses to phoneme recognition test speech signal to audiometer, to phones, to testor.
7. Testee's responses to phoneme recognition test speech signal to audiometer, to audio tape recorder.

The following measurements are made with warble tones and with live or recorded audio and audio-visual speech signals.

1 Obtain unaided warble-tone thresholds (250 Hz to 6000 Hz).

2 Obtain unaided speech reception threshold (SRT) using Select Spondiac Words (see Table 11). (Threshold = three words correct out of a sequence of five).

3 With live voice or tape recorded speech signal, obtain the most comfortable loudness level (MCL) using continuous sequence of Select Spondiac Words at a 45 dB hearing level (HL). Do this by having the client adjust gain of aid to most comfortable loudness level. To verify the MCL gain level setting of the aid, present the speech signal above and below 45 dB HL. Reset gain level of aid, if necessary, as needed for the best MCL level.

4 Obtain aided warble tone thresholds with aid set at MCL determined in Step 3. If the frequency-gain characteristics of the aid miss the Speech Spectrum Curve target, start over with another aid.

5 Obtain aided warble-tone threshold with aid set at full gain. If the difference between full gain setting and the MCL level is between 10 dB and 15 dB the aid will probably be worn by the user at the aid's reference test gain level. This will indicate that the aid has gain in reserve.

6 With aid set at full gain present Select Spondiac Words in a continuous sequence to obtain loudness discomfort level (LDL) of client. The LDL will determine the proper level of compression and the maximum output setting of the aid.

7 With aid set at MCL and speech level at 45 dB HL give either the Phoneme Recognition Quick Test or the Phoneme Recognition Inventory, depending upon the client's impairment. This will give some indication of the client's speech perception ability at about the intensity level of conversational speech. These phoneme recognition measurements may be made in quiet or in noise with a signal-to-noise ratio of + 5 dB.

If the speech level at 45 dB is too low for the client because of the severity of his hearing impairment, the speech signal should be raised to a level which will permit optimum phoneme recognition.

8 With speech signal set at the optimal intensity level (Step 7) present phoneme recognition test using another of the randomized lists of words with client watching speaker either live or through the VCR with TV screen directly above or below the loudspeaker.

Table 11
Select Spondiac Words*

1.	airplane	13.	dovetail	26.	eardrum	38.	dockyard
2.	foreword	14.	dogwood	27.	stairway	39.	wallboard
3.	greyhound	15.	earmark	28.	firebird	40.	glowworm
4.	hairbrush	16.	fireball	29.	earthworm	41.	downpour
5.	woodwork	17.	drawbridge	30.	foreward	42.	foolproof
6.	corkscrew	18.	cowboy	31.	downgrade	43.	daybreak
7.	sidewall	19.	railroad	32.	playground	44.	toothbrush
8.	doorway	20.	sailboat	33.	downfall	45.	foreworn
9.	schoolboy	21.	birthday	34.	trademark	46.	drumhead
10.	mousetrap	22.	hardware	35.	porthole	47.	doornob
11.	foreground	23.	baseball	36.	forescore	48.	forehead
12.	doorbell	24.	grapefruit	37.	armchair	49.	eyesore
		25.	proofread			50.	wholesale

*Spondiac words with a preponderance of vowels, semivowels and voiced consonants were selected for this list in order to avoid variability in intensity between words as occurs with words like "sunset" and "railroad". "Sunset" is relatively low in intensity as compared to "railroad" which is made up completely of voiced speech sounds. Consistency in intensity increases test validity and reliability and shortens testing time.

For obtaining the SRT use these words in the conventional manner. Three out of five words correct at a given intensity level is usually sufficient to establish the SRT. For obtaining the MCL and LDL use groups of five words, or more, in continuous sequence for each intensity level used in determining the MCL and LDL. We prefer this method for obtaining MCL and LDL over using pure tones or using a continuous speech message (often strangely referred to as "cold running speech") because we believe that it is more relevant and less time consuming than the above alternatives.

9 With the aided level of the SRT (Step 2) and the Phoneme Recognition loss (100% − score = loss) compute the Speech Perception Index (see Figure 8).

We hope that there will be hearing aid dispensers who will use some or all of the above steps, depending of course, upon the needs of the client and the circumstances of their practice. However, regardless of the hearing aid selection method the hearing aid dispenser uses, including computer-probe-tube-microphone ear canal measurements and quality judgements, they should bear in mind that the client's subjective auditory responses to amplification can, at least for the present, only be determined by means of true real-ear soundfield measurements.

THE SPEECH PERCEPTION INDEX

The intensity level of a person's speech reception threshold (SRT), and the extent of his phoneme recognition loss, give an indication of his ability to perceive speech. The utilization of this relationship was the objective of Hallowell Davis's Social Adequacy Index (1948). In spite of its good sense his index was never widely used. We have revived the concept and believe it is a logical way to measure the overall benefits of amplification for speech communication (Duffy 1967, 1984).

SPEECH PERCEPTION INDEX (SPI) *

Phoneme Recognition Loss (PRL)	Speech Reception Threshold (SRT)																	
	0	5	10	15	20	25	30	35	40	45	50	55	60	65	70	75	80	85
0	5	10	15	20	25	30	35	40	45	50	55	60	65	70	75	80	85	90
5	10	15	20	25	30	35	40	45	50	55	60	65	70	75	80	85	90	95
10	15	20	25	30	35	40	45	50	55	60	65	70	75	80	85	90	95	100
15	20	25	30	35	40	45	50	55	60	65	70	75	80	85	90	95	100	105
20	25	30	35	40	45	50	55	60	65	70	75	80	85	90	95	100	105	110
25	30	35	40	45	50	55	60	65	70	75	80	85	90	95	100	105	110	115
30	35	40	45	50	55	60	65	70	75	80	85	90	95	100	105	110	115	120
35	40	45	50	55	60	65	70	75	80	85	90	95	100	105	110	115	120	125
40	45	50	55	60	65	70	75	80	85	90	95	100	105	110	115	120	125	130
45	50	55	60	65	70	75	80	85	90	95	100	105	110	115	120	125	130	135
50	55	60	65	70	75	80	85	90	95	100	105	110	115	120	125	130	135	140
55	60	65	70	75	80	85	90	95	100	105	110	115	120	125	130	135	140	145
60	65	70	75	80	85	90	95	100	105	110	115	120	125	130	135	140	145	150
65	70	75	80	85	90	95	100	105	110	115	120	125	130	135	140	145	150	155
70	75	80	85	90	95	100	105	110	115	120	125	130	135	140	145	150	155	160
75	80	85	90	95	100	105	110	115	120	125	130	135	140	145	150	155	160	165
80	85	90	95	100	105	110	115	120	125	130	135	140	145	150	155	160	165	170
85	90	95	100	105	110	115	120	125	130	135	140	145	150	155	160	165	170	175

Impairment category labels within the table: *NORMAL*, *SLIGHTLY IMPAIRED*, *MODERATELY IMPAIRED*, *SEVERELY IMPAIRED*, *PROFOUNDLY IMPAIRED*.

Fig. 8.

To determine a person's Speech Perception Index (SPI) (see Figure 8) locate his speech reception threshold (SRT) at top (abscissa) and phoneme recognition loss (PRL) at side (ordinate). The number where the two lines intersect is the Speech Perception Index (SPI). The index is obtained with auditory and auditory-visual speech signals. The location of the index figure will indicate the client's degree of impairment, i.e., normal, slight, severe, profound.

EAR HYGIENE.

The glands that produce ear wax are situated in the outer one third to one half of the ear canal. Most types of earmolds or hearing aids occupy this area of the ear canal. When the aid is inserted, the wax often clings to the aid or mold or is pushed back into the ear canal. In addressing this matter we point out, on a diagram of the ear canal, the location of the wax glands, the same region of the ear canal to be occupied by the aid or earmold. We then describe a simple, safe, ear hygiene procedure as follows: With a cotton tipped applicator, with the cotton adjusted to be slightly smaller in diameter than the ear canal and moistened with a skin moistening lotion, gently ream out the outer wax-producing region of the ear canal being careful not to push the wax further into the ear canal. Do not use an unmoistened applicator for fear of irritating the ear canal. Repeat this procedure with clean, similarly moistened, applicators until the wax is removed. One or two repetitions are usually sufficient. The last application will leave the ear canal lubricated and the aid or mold will slide smoothly into place. Those persons who follow this procedure daily seldom have ear wax problems. With care not to place the applicator further into the ear canal than is necessary, that being the area usually occupied by the hearing aid or earmold, this procedure is harmless. Of course, if one has impacted wax which lies beyond the depth of the earmold or aid, a physician should remove it (Duffy 1986).

EAR IMPRESSIONS.

Although the syringe injection technique for making ear impressions is the most widely used method, it is not necessarily always the best. An alternative might be called the "spoon insertion method." I have found that for very tight molds for adults and especially for young children with soft, stretchable outer ears and ear canals, the spoon insertion method works best. Briefly, the procedure is as follows:

1 Inspect the ear canal with an otoscope and clean canal with a lotion lubricated cotton-tipped applicator.

2 Insert sponge block, attached to a string, as far into the ear canal as is needed for a proper fitting mold.

3 Mix only enough impression material to fill the ear canal and the lower portion of the concha. While the material is plastic and malleable, push and knead the material deep into ear canal with a smooth, blunt tipped, narrow ($1/4$ inch or less wide) metal spoon and pack against blocking plug. Without distorting the normal shape of the outer ear and ear canal, continue to knead the

material into the canal until its stiffness does not allow it to ooze out on either side of the spoon.

4 Without distorting the shape of the outer ear fill the concha and the remaining portion of the outer ear with a fresh batch of impression material. This material, while still soft, will weld itself to the canal portion of the impression.

5 Remove impression from ear when material has set.

Comment: The difference in size, when the syringe technique is compared with the spoon insertion method, is sometimes considerable, especially with small children.

HEARING REHABILITATION.

The procedures we have outlined are addressed to the hearing aid dispenser who will take the time to make a "good fit" rather than a "quick fit" that only "takes minutes" to perform. They will gain knowledge of the performance of a hearing aid as it relates to audibility for the client. They will gain knowledge of the phoneme recognition capability of the client for both auditory and auditory-visual speech signals.

With this information the hearing aid dispenser can advise the client and his family members regarding ways to improve auditory learning and to adjust to amplification in the home and at work.

The client and family members should be apprised of the significance of the client's place on the Speech Perception Index. They must learn of the client's potential for speech perception, they must be advised of accommodations to the client that they must make and they must be advised of ways in which the client can improve his auditory and auditory-visual perception of speech.

SUMMARY.

The client who initially finds amplified sounds disturbing must be encouraged to understand that the hearing aid which may, at first, make things sound strange and different, including speech, also makes it possible for him to hear sounds that he was unable to hear before. For these cases one must demonstrate to the client that with the hearing aid he can recognize words that he otherwise would miss. He must be assured that with auditory and auditory-visual learning his hearing aid will, before too long a time, sound "natural" to him. This is a point that is sadly missed by those who advocate a "quality judgement," "transparent" hearing aid selection procedure.

Most clients will appreciate the relatively short time it takes the hearing aid specialist to explain the significance of the results of the measurements made during the kind of hearing aid selection process we have described. Providing the client with proper amplification and advice which will be helpful to him is a proven way for the hearing aid dispenser to earn the confidence, respect and good will of the client.

THE LAST WORD.

Some years ago it was argued by some audiologists that hearing aids were only the beginning and not the end of hearing rehabilitation. They were going to change that.

Unfortunately, even after many new generations of hearing aid dispensers have entered the field, most of them with academic training in audiology, surprisingly little has changed. This, in spite of amazing advances in hearing aid technology.

In this chapter we have made an attempt to bridge the gap between hearing aid dispensing and hearing rehabilitation by describing procedures designed to discover the basic hearing communication potential and needs of the hearing-impaired person. It is this information which forms the basis for hearing rehabilitation.

GLOSSARY

Audiology The word literally means the study of audition. The study of audition and care for the hearing impaired did not begin, as some may believe, with those of us who participated in the U.S. Army's Aural rehabilitation Programs during World War II. The names of just a few of the notable "audiologists" who were in the field years before it received the name "audiology" include: R. A. Barlow; G. von Bekesy; A. G. Bell; C. C. Bunch; H. Davis; L. Dean; H. Fletcher; C. P. Fowler; S. F. Lybarger; S. Reger; J. C. Steinberg; S. S. Stevens; R. L. Wegel; A. M. Wengel; R. West.

Consonants Unvoiced consonants are the noise sounds of speech made from air escaping under pressure in a steady flow, as with fricatives, or when exploded, as with plosives. Voiced consonants combine the noises, described above for the unvoiced consonants, with the addition of phonation.

Earmold Occlusion Effect In pure-tone audiometric testing, measurements are made with the headphones occluding the ears. A hearing aid is selected which will compensate for the hearing loss portrayed by the client's audiogram. In the case of a client aided with an occluding earmold, a soundfield warble-tone test will measure the amplification provided by the aid as compared to the unaided soundfield measurement. Amplification restores occlusion loss. Loss of sound from the occlusion effect is seldom a significant factor in hearing aid selection.

Formant The overtones or harmonics of the fundamental tone are the formants. The lowest area of resonance constitutes the first formant with higher areas of resonance classified as second and third formants.

Frequency-Gain Characteristics The gain the hearing aid provides, from low frequencies to high frequencies, over the range of frequencies being amplified.

Fundamental Frequency The laryngeal tone produced by the vibrations of the vocal cords.

Phoneme A speech sound that is recognized as belonging to a family of sounds with acoustic characteristics which distinguish it from another phoneme, another speech sound family.

Real Genuine, actual, true, not deceptive.

Real-Ear Measurements Auditory responses which involve the entire hearing mechanism from the outer ear to the brain.

Speech Spectrum Curve The phonetic energy in the sounds of speech become increasingly weaker as the frequencies become higher. To compensate for this condition, we believe that the aided frequency-gain curve should gradually rise by 15 dB between 500 Hz and 4000 Hz. Speech sounds, to be perceived, must be heard at a supra-threshold level. Obviously, if these sounds are inaudible to the client they cannot be perceived.

Note: The frequency-gain response curves supplied by the manufacturers or from a hearing aid analyzer usually provide sufficient information for selecting aids which meet the speech spectrum curve target. The only way to find out if they do is through genuine real-ear soundfield measurements (see Figures 2, 3, 4).

Transition Frequencies The frequency changes which are made as one speech sound blends into another are called transition frequencies. These frequency changes, when recognized by the listener, often provide a clue to the end sound even though it may be inaudible.

Transparent If a high-fidelity audio system makes reproduced sound which is indistinguishable from the original input signal, in audio parlance, the output signal of the system is "transparent." The term has questionable application in hearing aid selection.

Vowels & Semivowels A voiced speech sound resonated and emitted through the mouth without any appreciable obstruction is called a vowel. Vowels made with the tongue arched toward the front of the mouth are called front vowels while vowels made with the tongue arched with the back part of the tongue are called back vowels. The vowel [u] as in "but" is made with the tongue relatively flat and is called a middle tongue vowel. Semivowels are vowel-like sounds that initiate, join, and terminate vowels, and are called "glides." In the case of [r] and [l] they also perform the function of vowels in the final syllable in words.

Warble-Tone Soundfield Audiometry A soundfield audiometric procedure for measuring the true real-ear responses of a client to warble tones without and with a hearing aid. It is a simple, practical procedure conducted with the most basic audiometric instrumentation. It does not involve conversion tables, calculations, formulae, or other theoretical manipulations of questionable validity and uncertain reliability.

REFERENCES.

BERGER, K. W. (1970): The Hearing Aid: Its Operation and Development, The National Hearing Society, Detroit, MI, p. 52.

DAVIS, H. (1948): The articulation area and the social adequacy index for hearing. *Laryngoscope*, Vol. 58, pp. 761-778.

DAVIS, H., STEVENS, S. S., NICHOLS, R. H., Jr., HUDGINS, C. V., MARQUIS, R. J., PETERSON, G. E., & ROSS, D. A. (1947): Hearing Aids, An Experimental Study of Design Objectives, Harvard University Press, Cambridge, Mass.

DUFFY, J. K. (1984): The role of phoneme-recognition audiometry in hearing rehabilitation. *The Hearing Journal*, Vol. 37, No. 4, pp. 24-29.

DUFFY, J. K. (1967): Audio-visual speech audiometry and a new audio-visual speech perception index. *Maico Audiological Library Series*, Vol. V, Report 9, pp. 1-3.

DUFFY, J. K. (1978): Sound field audiometry and hearing aid advisement. *Hearing Instruments*, Vol. 29, No. 2, pp. 6-12.

DUFFY, J. K. (1986): Book review. Ear and Hearing. Williams & Wilkins, Baltimore, MD, p. 116.

FLETCHER, H. (1953): Speech and Hearing in Communication, Van Nostrand Co., Princeton, NJ.

MARTIN, F. N., HAWKINS, R. R. & BAILEY, H. A. T. JR. (1962): The nonessentiality of the carrier phrase in phonetically balanced (PB) word testing. *J. Audit. Res.*, Vol. 2, pp. 319-322.

PETERSON, G. E. and BARNEY, H. L. (1952): Control methods used in a study of the vowels. *J. Acoust. Soc. Amer.*, 24, 175-184.

AUDIO AND VIDEO TAPES of the Phoneme Recognition Inventory and the Phoneme Recognition Quick Test are available from: Speech and Hearing Habilitation Films, Inc., 41 Amherst Road, Port Washington, NY 11050.

WEST, R., KENNEDY, L., & CARR, A. (1937): The Rehabilitation of Speech, Harper and Brothers, New York, NY, p. 159.

WEST, R., KENNEDY, L. & CARR, A. (1947): The Rehabilitation of Speech, Harper and Brothers, New York, NY, p. 559.

Subject Index